HEALING BEFORE YOU'RE CURED

The Evidence-based Guide to

Taking Control of Your Body and Mind

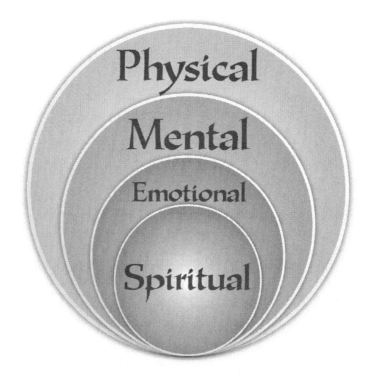

Roy Vongtama, MD

Resonant Books
A division of Resonant Entertainment LLC
www.resonantentertainment.com

Cover Design by Anurup Ghosh

ISBN: 978-0-9600033-0-3

Sign up to receive free tips and techniques on optimizing your health at www.MDRoy.com

TABLE OF CONTENTS

PREFACE

MY LIFE HAS BEEN a study in extremes.

Some contrasts are obvious and palpable–and made me *feel* different from birth. I grew up as one of the only Asian kids in a predominantly Caucasian town. I am almost 6′ 2″ and my parents are both a foot shorter than I am. I went to a Catholic school for 12 years even though our family is Buddhist.

Then there are those contrasts that are less obvious–but even more impactful. My father and mother, both Western-trained doctors, worked a lot– and that meant, as a child, I was often taken care of by someone other than my parents: a nanny, aunt, uncle, or grandmother. In addition, even though I was born in Buffalo, New York, my first language was Thai, not English, because Thai is what my grand-mother and nanny spoke. When I entered pre-kindergarten, my parents were told that if I continued speaking Thai, I would speak with an accent for the rest of my life- and so I spoke English from then on. As a result, every time some ignorant kid said, "Go back to China!" I would go "back" to *Thailand* in my mind, but I could neither speak nor really understand the language. I felt like an outsider everywhere I went.

Science and proof ruled my family–as my father, mother, and brother are all doctors. My dad was always very encouraging about my dreams, but with a very Asian caveat: "You can do whatever you want–*after* you finish

1

medical school!" Like a good son, I finished 21 years of school and became a medical doctor. This was widely celebrated by everyone around me but in my heart, I still felt like the same kid who didn't fit in. At least now I could rationalize that I had a few more letters to put after my name!

I found my way to Los Angeles by scoring an interview for residency training at UCLA. When the chairman [Fermi Award-winning[1]] H. Rodney Withers, asked me why I wanted to come to UCLA, I took a leap of faith and told him the truth: "I want to be an actor." And he shockingly replied, "I wanted to do that, too!" With a big sigh of relief (and a much-needed vote of confidence) I was offered residency at UCLA and spent four years there in radiation oncology training–all the while studying at night with some of the best acting coaches in the world.

At the end of my UCLA residency, I had a choice between acting in an indie movie or doing the rounds of interviews for a job as a full-time doctor. I chose the movie. (My mom didn't speak to me for months.) After the movie, I started to book roles in Hollywood (*The Shield*, *24*, *CSI*, and most notably, *The Bucket List* with Jack Nicholson and Morgan Freeman). Even though I was booking big projects, I found that in the bigger parts I would audition for, I was getting a lukewarm reception at best, sometimes because I was Asian and they couldn't see me outside of a stereotype but also because of something that was missing inside of me. I couldn't figure what that missing thing was, but thankfully one of my early acting coaches, Carolyne Barry (who has

1 The Fermi Award is one of the highest scientific awards in the world and is presented for lifetime achievement in the field of the development use of energy. Dr. Withers won in 1996.

since passed because of cancer), brought this situation to a head. She used to have me get up and say my name. I would get up, smile and say, "Roy Vongtama?" She would just look at me and say, "Is that a statement or a question?" I would answer, "A statement?" And then she would say, "Nope. Sit down." This went on for a few weeks, me, standing up, saying "Roy Vongtama?" and then being told to sit down. I became very frustrated, as I felt like wasn't learning anything about acting. I was just getting up and being told to say my name, and then getting told to sit down in front of the rest of the class! The last time it happened, I was visibly angry. Carolyne asked me, "Why would a handsome, smart guy like you not know how to say his name?" I snorted a reply, "I don't know." She asked me, "Wait. Are you saying you don't know *why* you don't know how to say your name, or you don't know that you're attractive?" I said, "I don't know." She turned to the class, which on that day was mostly female. She asked them, "Who here agrees with me?" They all raised their hands. I snorted again. "They *have* to say that, you're the teacher." She just looked at me, and said, "Wow. You think *everyone* is lying to you? You don't need acting class. You need therapy." I left that night feeling so angry. I couldn't believe she had embarrassed me like that in front of everyone. After a couple hours passed when I had calmed down, I asked a better question: "Why don't I believe them?" I didn't know, but I knew that something was wrong. Seriously wrong. I had to figure this out- I had to figure *me* out. I needed to be able to take in what other people were saying to me and letting that be real, or at least try it on for size. That's how acting works, as Sanford Meisner, the great acting coach, said: "Acting is reacting."

My sole focus then became about *knowing myself*: through therapy, meditation, journaling, and of course, acting classes.

This story, though, isn't all about my acting career and me. Somewhere along my inward journey, something very interesting and profound happened on the "other side" of my dual career paths. Because of all the work I was doing to figure myself out for the sake of my acting career, I had become something even more rare than an actor who knows how to listen. I had become a *doctor* who knows how to listen. I could *connect* with patients. I could hear their deeper needs and respond with authentic caring, because I could *feel* how they felt. I also started to counsel my patients on the benefits of positive thinking, emotional work, and meditation–sometimes discussing and teaching all three subjects in one session. Patients today, perhaps feeling heard for the first time, still ask me curiously, "What school did you say you went to?"

I share with you all of this background information so you can understand my unique perspective and why I feel it's so important to look outside the box–and why I feel that taking real and permanent ownership of your health is what true healing is all about.

INTRODUCTION

"All truth passes through three stages. First, it is ridiculed. Second, it is violently opposed. Third, it is accepted as being self-evident."

- often attributed to Arthur Schopenhauer,
a German philosopher

Maybe because I lived for so long in a place without integrity, then moved to a place inside myself with high integrity, I am now acutely aware what both spaces feel like. My antennae go up when I feel something is being sold as "the solution"–particularly when it clearly is false. With the advent of direct marketing of drugs, the rise of processed foods as the main staple of nutrition, and the overuse of the medical quick fix in the American health consciousness, the voice of what really is healthy has been drowned out. *My goal in this book is to connect you back to health, using not just my own knowledge–and not just common sense–but* real *science*.

I avoided writing this book for many years because I was concerned about the repercussions from the Western medical establishment–as I am a member of that community.

I've let that concern go. I now feel it is more important to give a voice to the power of a balanced approach to health, and if I come under criticism for it, then so be it.

Many of my physician friends often are very excited about what I am talking and writing about–because they also realize that much of what I speak of is necessary, not just in their patients' lives, but in their own as well. We, doctors and patients alike, simply have not been taught what "healthy" really means.

We take an oath when we become doctors "to do no harm." But sadly, many doctors will react negatively when they hear a patient is trying something outside the Western norm. This reaction doesn't come from a scientific exploration of the evidence, but just good old-fashioned ignorance. "It doesn't matter what you eat," cancer patients tell me their other doctors have informed them. Nutrition doesn't matter if you practice "ignorance is bliss." But if you really are looking for the truth, you'll see that it does matter and matters a great deal.

The good news is that a wholly integrated approach is synergistic, meaning it works in combination, with what Western medicine provides. Notice I used the term "wholly integrated" and did not write *alternative* or *complementary*, which is what most Western doctors would call it. Those terms imply that non-Western approaches are merely add-ons, as if they were not important. This arrogance by close-minded Western doctors often makes patients feel like their own efforts to educate themselves on different approaches (and to take control of their own health) are insignificant.

I am convinced that what we can do with our personal choices *before* we get sick is as important (if not more important) than almost every choice we make *after* we get sick. Most of what I will present in this book shows you that the body can, and does, heal *itself, before* and *after* diagnosis–*given your own personal reinforcement and support.*

On the other hand, I am still a Western-trained doctor and I believe Western medicine has a significant place in health. There are radical, holistic voices tweeting and blogging that Western medicine is a sham. I have heard more than once about "the conspiracy" behind Western medicine. There is no conspiracy. Just look at the results of cancer treatments today. We are curing 65 percent of malignant cases (ones that if left untreated would cause eventual death or morbidity). This represents a 22 percent rise in cure rates over the last 20 years[i] and amounts to almost 200,000 more lives saved per year than 20 years ago!

I do believe, however, that 6,000 years of holistic experience from the East can be balanced effectively with $6 trillion dollars of research from the West. After reading this book, I hope that you will agree with me. This idea of combining both sides is where the title of the book came from. "Healing" is a process that we accomplish from the *inside*, which is the focus of the Eastern holistic approach. "Curing" is a process that comes from the *outside*, which is the focus of the Western approach. I believe both are useful, but healing places the control within you, whereas curing usually requires something or someone else to get you back to health.

How Did This Book Come to Be?

Why would I write a book that looked to combine the physical, mental, emotional, and spiritual into one paradigm? I am a Western-trained doctor – so why not just follow the party line?

As I mentioned in the preface, I grew up in a Buddhist family and went to Catholic school until I was 18 years old. I had many "instructions" to follow from both home and school and as a result, I became very suspicious about following other people's rules and regulations. In fact, in my junior year of Jesuit high school, I asked to be removed from religion class. When the priest asked me why, I replied that I wanted to search for answers myself, because I wasn't finding any in class.

To the Jesuits' credit, I was granted independent study five days a week. I was excited because, as a 16-year-old, I got to skip religion class every day! The only part I hadn't counted on was that I had to do a book report on a new topic every week! But these mandatory assignments led me to research many interesting topics that opened my mind to the possibility that the answers are almost always out there somewhere. Now, whenever I ask myself, "Why?", I am confident that I can find the answer. I just have to keep looking.

All through my adolescence, my parents stressed the importance of eating right, getting enough sleep, and exercise. This "training" is the basis for what you will find in the *Physical House* section of this book. My understanding of "eating right" is different from what my mom's definition is (imagine heated family discussions over the importance of eating beef-my mom's favorite meat) but the fact that they stressed good nutrition is imprinted in my mind.

When I entered the University of Pennsylvania as an undergraduate, I was identified as someone who might be susceptible to depression, based on a pre-entrance test I had taken. I was asked to participate in a study that taught freshmen how to critically analyze our thoughts, which the investigators thought would help us prevent and cope with depression (should it choose to rear its ugly head). This idea that changing your thoughts could lead to wellness became the basis for the positive psychology movement that has emerged over the last 20 years. I have used the skills that I learned in college, and over the years have expanded on them. I have witnessed in my own life just how powerful utilizing positive, life-affirming thoughts can be as part of a good health practice. Thus, was born the *Mental House* section of this book.

My parents were both abandoned as children and never dealt with their traumas in a direct way. I lived in a home where emotional safety was not of paramount concern and where, if I did what I was told, I would be relatively safe from criticism and judgment. This led to a profound inability to express my emotions in a healthy way. Ironically, this lack of emotional well-being led me to acting, where emotions and behavior are the tools of the trade. Not surprisingly, I wasn't a very good actor! When I started taking acting classes at night during medical training, I was told the classic line: "Maybe you should keep your day job." But being that I have always been ultra-competitive, I took that comment about my [lack of] talent as motivation to go deeper into acting.

I also did eventually take the advice to go to therapy to deal with my "stuck" emotions. (I didn't even know emotions could get stuck!) Over time, working with a therapist helped me dramatically improve my physical and emotional health, not to mention my overall happiness and sense of well-being. These transforming results became the genesis for the *Emotional House* section.

The *Spiritual House* ties everything together. During my early years in Los Angeles, I had become relatively successful both as an actor and as a Board-Certified radiation oncologist. From the outside looking in, I had all the trappings of prosperity and achievement. It should have amounted to my feeling happy and content. However, I was anything but. I just could not see my life as successful at all.

I knew I needed to search again, to go deeper inside, just as I had in high school and after medical school.

One day, after some cajoling, a friend brought me to a meditation center called Lake Shrine, in Pacific Palisades, CA, and after a healthy dose of skepticism, I finally tried meditation.

At first, I could meditate for about 60 seconds before I had to get up and move. Being as how I never allow myself to fail at anything though (thanks again Mom and Dad!) I kept at it. It wasn't easy but it was worth it. Having kept my meditation practice for many years now and seeing how much meditation has improved my happiness and overall life, I know it has to serve as a keystone in any thriving formula for health.

The bottom line is that all of the Houses—Physical, Mental, Emotional, and Spiritual– are critically important to your overall health and well-being. The key is to take ownership of each area, empowering yourself to change. I did -- and I know for certain that you can too.

TAKING OWNERSHIP

This book is nothing but words bundled into pages made from dead trees. That is, this book is a waste if the only thing you do with it is READ the pages.

Instead, I would like you to read this book—and then allow the words and paragraphs and chapters to change you.

Allow the contents to permeate your life.

Embrace the information in this book and try some of the things out, experiment with them, create a relationship with them.

Like any relationship, if they work for you, keep them, and if they do not work, then move on.

The Holy Grail of Medicine

A doctor's goal in deciphering a person's illness is to find a <u>unifying diagnosis</u>: *One* overarching reason for why the illness happened. I am the son of two doctors—I grew up immersed in medical discussions—and I was always struck by how many diagnoses, based on accepted scientific thinking, were often so regimented and segmented. For example, I would hear my mom say, "Justin's dad has really bad asthma, and needs to see a doctor." So, Justin's dad would go to a lung specialist (AFTER seeing his primary care doctor first). Later, when Justin's dad got migraines, he had to go see a totally different doctor, a neurologist, to get a remedy for the migraines. At that visit, the asthma wouldn't even be talked about, as it wasn't in the same "system." After hearing repeated stories like this, I often wondered, "Could these two seemingly separate things be related? Couldn't ONE reason be the cause for both?" But I never heard that sort of thinking even considered in medical school.

Just as often I would hear about patients with a disease, for example, breast cancer, treated with familiar processes, such as surgery and radiation, in the hope that the treatment would result in a "cure." The treatment, often resulted in a very happy patient who was "back to normal" (meaning, in reality, no longer in the extreme disease state) but the *cause* of the disease was never *really found* or *even considered.* The most that would be discussed would be the role of risk factors, genetics, and family history, but this discussion would be maximally 1 minute out of an hour's meeting. My curiosity led me to ask myself, "Besides genetics, what allowed her to get breast cancer? Did her terrible eating habits contribute? Did her super high stress level affect it? What about her negative thinking?" These questions, again, seemed not along the lines of thought taught in medical school.

The root cause of disease is so often not found because Western-trained doctors have often not had the training (nor sometimes the inclination) to look beyond what is currently provable. If you ask a doctor why someone got cancer, you will hear predictable answers about genetics, behavioral risk factors, and exposures. But these aren't really the causes of the cancer! These are simply signposts that popped up *after* a person was diagnosed. If genetics and risk factors and exposures were foolproof predictors, then we could theoretically all adhere to doctor-approved recommend-dations in order to *avoid* cancer. As a doctor, I could say, "You have this gene. You have this risk factor. With this exposure you will get cancer." We know though that such predictions are not infallible. We all know many people who have the worst habits and exposures and family history of cancer—but they don't get cancer. And we all know people with the best diet and physical fitness regimens who still, for one reason or another, do get cancer.

What does this mean? We know that the causes of cancer *aren't always* clear. The causes of cancer are far more encompassing than just clinical markers and behavioral signposts. So, what should we be looking for?

We should not be searching for the all-encompassing, unifying diagnosis or reason. Instead we should seek a unifying perspective, a unifying approach that cancer can be seen through and thus treated successfully.

Another way to look at the word "diagnosis" is that it is a term used to label a set of symptoms and signs that gives us a framework of understanding. This understanding has associated treatments that hopefully cure the diagnosis. This works great when a high cure rate is achievable. However, what if that diagnosis does *not* have a treatment that leads to a cure? If there is no cure or no effective treatment, then the diagnosis, which ultimately is simply a word, actually becomes detrimental. The diagnosis then makes everyone, including the doctor, believe that nothing can be done.

If the lens is adjusted to take the focus off of the diagnosis and look instead with a broader perspective, *then the focus is removed from what we cannot do and placed onto what we can do.* In fact, through this enlarged scope, we can accurately see ALL diseases and treat from this perspective.

There are many diseases, but only one health.

What do I mean by only "one health"? What I mean is that regardless of what diagnoses you have been given, what symptoms you have, the goal we are all trying to reach is the same: health. And that health is universal. This also implies that our bodies will *always* respond towards health when given the chance, if we have taken the time to listen to it. The best part is that with this unifying perspective, this "one health," we can actually *see* much earlier where a person is off balance and try to bring the person back to health *before* something irrevocable happens, like a cancer diagnosis.

An Analogy: Your Body as a Car

Imagine that your body is a car. When it doesn't start, a lot of thoughts and emotions go through us: "How will I get to work? How much will it cost? I hope it's not the engine," and on and on. We all have had the anxiety and feeling the fear of the unknown this situation brings.

The good news is that the car will be running again with the expertise of an amazing mechanic. Eventually the car comes back to you, not good as new maybe, but it runs again. The question is: Who is now responsible for keeping the car running well? Is it *only* the mechanic's job? Of course not. We are responsible for it, because we own it. Unfortunately, many of us do expect "one stop at the shop" will keep the car running forever.

In much the same way, too many of us expect our doctors to pick anything and everything up in the increasingly common fifteen-minute visit. In older times, doctors had longer visits, got to know their patients a lot better over time, and even made house calls, which really would give a doctor an insight into a person's well-being. Nowadays, insurance and hospitals make the call as to how long a patient is seen. Even with this being mostly common knowledge, we still expect that the roadmap will be clearly laid out for us after being treated for a disease, especially after a staggering diagnosis like cancer. There is definitely more time spent before a treatment starts, but after the treatment is over, as you or a loved one may have found out, "getting a roadmap" isn't what happens. Doctors will just watch to make sure nothing is wrong, by getting scans and lab tests. It's more like a waiting game, or as we call it in medicine: "watchful waiting," or "active surveillance."

That's not good enough for me, and it shouldn't be for you either. There's more that can be done, and that's what you will learn in this book. We'll look at physical, mental, emotional and spiritual techniques that will make you an active participant in your own health.

If you're like most people, the prospect of doing it all yourself is scary and may not even be possible, and that's not what I am suggesting. What I am talking about is taking ownership of the decisions, given the choices you have in front of you. Why must it be you? Think about it: Who truly is responsible for your body—what you eat, when you exercise, how you engage spiritual guidance? YOU!

Most of us would like someone else—a doctor, a therapist, a priest—to make decisions and to offer specific advice and counsel. Why? We believe finding the right physical, mental, emotional, and spiritual path is too difficult and is often too overwhelming. Plain and simple, most of us like to take the easy path.

Unfortunately, the easy path isn't always the best path.

Throughout this book I relate my experiences with people and patients that I've encountered. My goal is to provide personal perspectives and help you to see that this integrated approach really works!

Larry had throat cancer. Sometimes with older patients, especially men, I try to liken their body to that of their first car. I try to get them to remember how special it was to ride in. Many people (not just men!) have had that kind of experience: the power they felt when driving it, the freedom, and especially the joy. It gets them excited about going through the long process of healing. In this case, Larry had a 1955 Thunderbird. Larry said, "That sounds great! I can't wait to get back to that new car!" The truth, though, is that Larry can't go back—the shiny new car isn't around anymore. What I reminded Larry was this: "You know, you can't go back, but you know what you can be? <u>The remodeled *refurbished classic,*</u> which is oftentimes *more valuable* than the original!"

In that same way, we have to be enthusiastic about what health we can achieve *now,* in this current body, and guess what, you never know, you might feel better than you ever did before.

Taking Ownership of Your Health
(Yes, I am repeating myself!)

This analogy of a car and your body is all about you taking ownership of your health and your life. Our culture has shifted from one where we received information from respected experts who could be trusted to one in which all the information is at your fingertips (through the internet, etc.). Even more so, experts seem to be something to be scoffed at. Certainly, there are advantages to having information easily accessible, but we need to proceed with some caution.

As an example, I got into a Facebook argument with a health industry friend about a scientific issue and she posted a blog as part of her "proof," which I clicked on and quickly found out was written by a 19-year-old girl who hadn't gone to college nor had been trained in any scientific thought process. Not only was it *not* a scientific journal, but the girl writing the blog wasn't even trained in anything!

My point in relating this story is that too often, we only look for evidence that supports something we already believe. (This is called *confirmation bias.*) We rarely look for evidence to find what is true and what is not, which would be more helpful to us. Why is this? I believe it is because if we had to actually admit to ourselves that something we did was not good for us, we would have to at least consider changing. And human beings do not like to change!

What I say to people who come to me for health advice is to at least *hear* what the information is. No one is going to force you to do anything. As my mentor from UCLA, Dr. Guy Juillard, who was the Vice Chair of UCLA Radiation Oncology, said to patients who were unsure whether they wanted a treatment or not: "We can't treat you without you." Basically, he was saying we won't do anything without your permission and more importantly, make sure you are on board with whatever treatment you decide on. *So, in short, make a vow to yourself that you are in charge.* Interestingly, whenever Dr. Juillard would say this, with a rare exception patients would take ownership and commit to treatment.

The first step is learning what you can do on your own, seeing if it resonates with you, and if it doesn't, discard it. The second step is to enlist experts whom you trust that have knowledge in areas that you need to grow in, whether by books, videos or in person. I have personally received many of these calls from friends and relatives. I understand the fear of burdening an expert friend with unwanted trouble, but personally I am grateful to be of service but also am happy they took the opportunity to be vulnerable and ask for help. So, take a chance, and don't let your fear be the reason you don't ask for help. You're still the boss!

The Four Houses of Health

The Four Houses of Health–physical, mental, emotional and spiritual–is the framework that I use for teaching patients about the paradigm of wellness.

If we break down how most people think about health, the Four Houses look something like this:

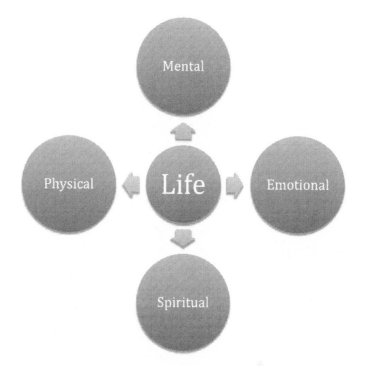

This is a very compartmentalized view of health. Most people approach their lives in this same segregated manner, and in some regards, there is a certain simplicity to this way of living. It is also true that the medical establishment (and society in general) encourages this separateness, causing each House to appear independent of each other.

In our daily lives, each problem we face requires a specialist in one form or another. If we have a spiritual issue, we go to our rabbis, priests or pastors. If we have a mental issue, we seek guidance from our therapists or counselors. And if we have a physical problem, we head to our doctors. For example:

1. You break a bone.
2. The doctor sets the bone.
3. The bone heals in a cast.
4. The bone is back to normal.

This pattern is generally how we address disease and illness in the Western world. And although this formula appears to work, it operates only on the surface and is missing a lot of detail. The following case study will illustrate just how much more complex a health issue can be (and generally is).

Ray* is an annual volunteer at a weeklong summer camp for kids. His main job is to supervise the children and to help maintain their safety as they "play hard" during sports and activities. But Ray is an energetic leader (and a bit of a competitive athlete) so he can't help himself from joining in enthusiastically with the kids.

On the very first day of camp, Ray smacks his face directly into a telephone pole and needs superglue to keep the cut on his face from bleeding. Then the next day, he dislocates his shoulder playing water polo. On the advice of one of the camp leaders, Ray goes to see the yoga instructor, Norman, who has been known to help relieve injuries using certain yoga methods. As Norman works on him, Ray's shoulder begins to feel better.

"I always get hurt when I compete," Ray remarks almost proudly. "I've dislocated my shoulder five times, broke my ankle, tore my knee up, broke toes and have countless sprains and cuts."

Norman pauses, stares at Ray for a moment and then asks, "What are you gaining by getting hurt?"

Ray stares back at Norman, somewhat shocked. Ray had never really thought about this before, certainly not that there might be some "positive" reason why, for most of his life, he has repeatedly injured himself while competing.

While contemplating this new perspective, Ray remembers something from his past and then it all clicks for him. He recalls that as a child, his mother was only really nurturing to him and only physically cared for him *when Ray was injured.*

Putting the pieces together, Ray suddenly recognizes that unconsciously, he had played every sport, every event, with not just the intent to win but also to get hurt if he couldn't win. This had set up an ostensibly "win-win" situation for Ray: *approval* if he did win, or *affection* if he didn't.

So, from this example, you can see that there was a shoulder injury and it got better. The initial story could have ended there. But Norman was astute enough to consider the layers behind the physical. And Ray was receptive enough to be able to incorporate a more holistic view of the mental, the emotional and the spiritual aspects of health.

(*Full disclosure: The "Ray" in the story is me!)

Through this anecdote, we can *begin* to see what true healing really is:

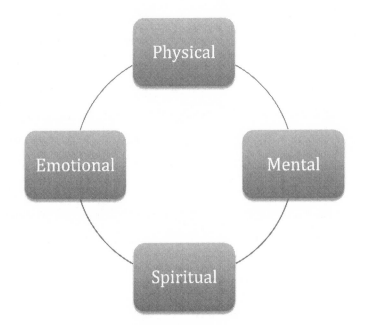

So, the first thing that we can infer from this more integrated approach to wellness is that all the "Houses of Health" are connected and interconnected. That may now seem pretty obvious, in light of the above example, but how many people approach their lives with this knowledge?

From my years of experience with patients, and in my own life in general, I have found that there are very few (maybe about 5%) who have awareness of the links between the physical, mental, emotional and spiritual aspects of health. And of those with this cognizance, maybe only half actively apply this wisdom in their lives.

Yet, it is within the awareness, the consciousness of interconnectedness, that health lies. Accepting this interdependence as truth is where health needs to *start* not end. When we do this, both subtle and profound changes can begin to take place in our personal and collective health.

An important point for all of us to understand about interconnectedness is that if a person has a problem in one house and it is not dealt with within that house, *it will begin to cause problems in another.* When I go to treat a person who is physically sick, I do, of course, address the Physical House first: The bone needs to be set and a cast needs to be put on. However, as I am addressing the physical, I have also been trained by my experience to look at the other three houses simultaneously. For me, the Four Houses do not just connect; they are *intimately* related:

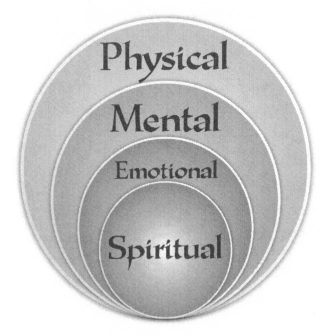

The above diagram shows us how closely related they are. Why is this so significant?

As an example, let's look at my specialty as an oncologist. Western medicine currently attacks cancer with only the weapons of the Physical House. To approach this devastating disease with only the tools from the Physical House is using only 25% of what is available to us. Why fight "the war on cancer" with only one quarter of what's available? It makes no sense. And the results of this mentality have played out unfortunately with catastrophic results in many cases.

Cancer is Not Solely a Biological Disease

For our purposes, let's define cancer how most people who are familiar with it might define it:

"Cancer is a disease in which a cell has gone bad–it's mutated to the point where it multiplies uncontrollably and if left untreated causes the body to die because the uncontrolled cells either reach a vital organ or overwhelm the entire system."

This is a fairly accurate *description* of cancer but the *definition* is incomplete. Even if I explained to you the genetic aberrations behind the development of cancer and the mutations that take place due to the environment, this still wouldn't make the definition complete. It might explain the *mechanism* but it would not explain *why* one person gets cancer and another does not.

Let me restate this for clarity. Two people can have the exact same genetic structure, with the same mutations and be exposed to the exact same environment and stressors, and one person may get cancer and the other may not. These mechanisms do not elucidate the "why." They simply tell us the "how." And the *how* is not enough.

So, what does this mean in actual practice for someone who is hoping to become healthy and is looking to stop a potential cancer or cancer recurrence?

It means that most people are missing a *major* link that stops people from being healthy: the connection between the mental, emotional and spiritual to the physical. It means that these *unseen* layers of life, very often painful to confront, have a very significant role to play in health.

The work of spiritual Japanese Artist/Author Masuro Emoto is fascinating to look at from this perspective. Trained at Open International University for Alternative Medicine, he has photographed water at freezing temperatures being affected by emotional states. He had participants enter different emotional states, e.g., hate versus love, had those people touch water in those states, and then photographed the effect on the pattern of crystallization when the water approached freezing. What he showed is that hate and anger had a crystallization pattern that was unordered and chaotic. On the other end, the crystallization of water from people feeling love was ordered and beautiful. When one thinks of the body and its composition being about 60-70% water, we start to see how things we cannot see like emotions can have an effect on the health of the body. (This isn't "proof" per se, but rather a small illustration of what we do not know regarding the interconnectedness of our Houses.)

Using Your Intuition

In general, people do not read science to learn, they read it to validate what they already believe. And when that science doesn't fit what they believe, they throw it out.

Of course, trained scientists are justifiably up in arms over the use of this artistic work as "evidence."

In an effort to make the cynics and actually, the scientific skeptic in me, comfortable, throughout this book I will give dozens of citations from peer-reviewed scientific journals to give some credibility to what I am presenting. However, that won't be enough for the skeptic, those who seemingly judge everything to prevent anything new (and possibly better) from actually landing inside their beings.

Here's the thing though that the skeptic misses: I don't *want* you to simply believe me. Keep reading and listen to what you *feel* about it. If you use *your own* intuition (your own gut feeling) to listen with, you will instinctively know what is true and what is not. This intuitive voice is the one that each of us must learn to listen to and to trust if we are to become healthier human beings.

The body *wants* to heal. If given the chance, that's just what it does.

One of the wonderful things about intuition is that it will always speak for what is best for you. The difficult part is that one has to continually and consistently practice listening to it in order to hear it. As you read this, you might find that the idea of listening to and trusting your intuition is too unbelievable or unachievable or too "out there." That's ok, because I'm not asking you to believe. I am asking you to be scientific- test it out! Try using that quiet, steady, assured, intuitive voice in low-risk, everyday situations (when, for example, you have two choices for a meal and there is no logical/obvious choice) and you'll begin to discover that it *always* guides you without fail to the answer that is best for you. That's real *experiential* "science" that's practical and applicable to every situation in your life.

What is interesting in my own life is that when I started to listen to my intuition, I realized there were *two* voices speaking up: one was my actual intuition and the other was my old friend, whom I might call "the protector" (or oftentimes "the terrorist") or what some psychologists would simply call, "the ego."

The problem that I found is that the "protector" often *seemed* to be giving me solid, really practical advice like, "make sure your business partners don't take advantage of you" or "you better eat fast because you might not have time to finish." But what I discovered was that my thoughts were making me *scared* and I was reacting to these thoughts out of fear rather than experiencing what was actually happening. In essence, I was distorting my reality in a way that *seemed* protective and self-preserving but in truth was based in anxiety and disquiet.

In each example above, I had to break down what was "actually" happening:

In the first example, "make sure your business partners don't take advantage of you," my business partners and I had a contract. Why should I assume that they would try to take advantage of me? I had no evidence of this. In fact, that's why I partnered with them, because I felt I could trust them. And even in the worst-case scenario, I was protected by the mutually signed contract. My mind was causing me to enter a state of fear unnecessarily.

In the second example, "you better eat fast because you might not have time to finish," I actually had plenty of time to eat. Why was I rushing? Was I reacting to the facts of the present moment or to some past fear regarding food?

So, I began to pay closer attention to my thoughts and to try to listen to that steady, quiet voice beneath the noise of fear and worry: My intuition.

Please don't feel like you are alone in feeling like this is a *huge* task. In the beginning, I found this constant delineation between my fear-based thoughts and my intuition to be often confusing (which voice is which?), humbling (because I thought I was making good decisions) and frustrating (maybe it's easier to just keep doing what I have always done).

The best advice I have ever received to discern whether it is my ego that is speaking or whether it is truly my intuition, was from a monk who had been one for at least 30 years. He told me, *"The intuitive voice speaks when you are calm. The voice of the ego speaks when you are in fear."*

(Just to remind us, when he was using the term "ego," the monk meant that part of our mind that is responsible for our self-identity and also regulates our perception of reality.)

If you look at both examples again, "make sure your business partners don't take advantage of you" and "you better eat that fast because you might not have time to finish," on the surface, they both appear to come from a place of practical concern. But in my actual experience, in my body, what I am feeling is *fear*. And that means that the ego is in charge, not my intuition. So even though it may feel even scarier to dismiss the "advice," since it arises from fear, it cannot be right for me *at that time*. If, on the other hand, later on when I was calm, a voice told me, "I don't know if I trust these guys..." and that voice did not generate fear, then I would have to take more time to listen to it, because that would likely be my intuition speaking up.

The bottom line is that each one of us knows that fear can be very powerful, persuasive and emotionally debilitating. But it can also be *physically* destructive. We will explore later in detail the mental-physical connection (popularly called the Mind-Body connection) in the Mental House, but to be clear: what you think and what you choose to continue thinking *does* directly (through DNA damage) and indirectly (through continued poor habits) affect our physical health. If we continue to allow this insidious voice to dictate to our minds what actions we must take, then we will be reinforcing the disease that has manifested in our lives.

Even look at the word: "Dis-ease." Broken down into its etymological roots: "Dis" means "a lack of" and "ease" is defined as "the state of being comfortable, or a feeling of freedom." The word itself holds the very thing that we need to fix it: a sense of ease, comfort and a feeling of freedom. Isn't this what health should feel like?

"Natural forces within us are the true healers of disease."

- Hippocrates

Your Life as Energy

Think of your body as a system, one that can release and absorb energy. This can come in the form of physical energy (like a hug or a punch), emotional energy (like love or anger), mental energy (like positive or negative thoughts) or spiritual energy (like a feeling of connectedness or disconnectedness).

When you, as a living organism, take in an experience, it registers in your body. By letting yourself feel the experience, something magical happens: the flow of energy happens naturally–the energy leaves your body. However, when you take in an experience and do not let it register (by pretending it didn't happen or pretending it didn't hurt you), you create a blockage, an impediment to flow. The natural instinctive release of energy is short-circuited. Unfortunately, most people take the second route. More-over, it gets compounded: we often avoid putting ourselves into that situation in an attempt consciously or un-consciously to protect ourselves from reliving or repeating that event. Had we simply FELT it, and let it flow through, yes it would have been painful, but it would have been part of the *past*. By letting it reside in our bodies, sometimes for years and even decades, it remains part of our *present*. Tragically, this path, on an energetic level, creates disease.

To make the point even clearer, let's break it down. If something happened to you when you were a child that caused you significant emotional pain, for instance, your

mother or father abandoning you (physically or emotionally), but you never mourned that loss, never expressed
the anger, grief and/or deep sorrow that you felt for being
abandoned, then what does that become? Does it simply go
away? From my experience, it only goes away if we take
time to understand it, to *look* at it, to become aware of what
is going on inside us. Most of the time though, the easier
path is to wall it off and pretend like it never happened.
Then we are sometimes not even consciously aware of that
anger, sadness, or pain.

As humans, we then project these negative feelings onto
the people and world around us, and we draw to ourselves
similar situations and people over and over again, replaying
out the same trauma. Like a pressure cooker, this oft-
repeated pattern continues to build negative energy because
there has been no healthy outlet for release. We fear that to
take the lid off this pot of pent up energy would cause us to
destroy ourselves by forcing us to experience these extraordinarily painful feelings all over again. But paradoxically,
it is this very fear of release that increases the power of this
negative energy to hurt us from the inside out. Because
regardless of our feelings about it, this trapped energy *must*
be freed. It *must* be expressed. It *has to* go somewhere.

So, for years upon years, we expend tremendous
amounts of vitality to keep this energy from coming out,
protecting ourselves by constantly staying on the go or
taking care of others instead of ourselves. What happens is
that eventually and inevitably, because everything is

connected (the physical to the mental to the emotional to the spiritual, and each to each other) this trapped energy manifests into malady. And this can take a number of different forms in the body from depression to disease to personality disorders and beyond. Taking our abandonment example from above, the hurt and rage and grief that results from a parent's neglect can sometimes physically manifest as cancer.

Does "resentment causes cancer" sound far-fetched to you? Think about what cancer does and how it behaves. A living, growing mass that *used to be normal* changes into something that violates the boundaries of other organs, doesn't care about the body it needs to live in, and spreads until it occupies the whole body until eventually, it kills the body and itself. Sounds a lot like "rage," doesn't it? Perhaps, not unlike how one might feel and behave if given the chance to express their losses, pain and suffering.

So, now that we see how compartmentalized energy inside us turns further inward and attacks in a variety of destructive ways, what can we do about it?

The key to healing is to recognize that although that energy must come out, we have the ability to choose the way it comes out.

Start journaling. Start therapy. See not just the external journey of life but the internal voyage. Discover the feelings you are holding inside. Dive deeper into the events you are holding onto. Express your emotions.

And one of the most potent tools that you already have in your arsenal is the power of forgiveness. Forgive yourself for the burden you have been carrying since you were a child. Forgive yourself for not dealing with it sooner. Forgive those who have wounded you, for that is what resentment is: non-forgiveness for a hurt that happened in the past. Easier said than done right? Don't worry. We'll get more into the "how" in the *Emotional House* section.

Ever since I was young, I have always been fascinated with behavioral patterns and looked for them everywhere. It made me a proficient scientist and also a pretty good predictor of behavior. When I decided to use my ability to see patterns to look in the mirror, this skill set humbled me. I saw a lot of patterns that needed to change, but with some courage, it became a very productive tool for self-improvement.

To discover what deeply held feelings I had from the past, I looked at what present events in my life triggered resentment. Try it. If you are harboring resentments against people and situations currently in your life, they will most likely be shadows of old resentments from long past. Look for the patterns. Are there situations and relationships that keep appearing again and again? Is there something you are meant to learn from them?

There is a saying that a friend related to me, which I like very much: "Every third person is your teacher." The meaning behind it is that every person we meet can offer us a potentially life-changing lesson. It's up to us to be open enough and aware enough to see what that lesson may be. (And for me personally, if every third person is supposed to be my teacher, then I haven't really been paying attention!)

A classic example: The Annoying Employee at Work. Why does that person at work annoy us so much? Typically, we look at their behavior and we judge them. We might say something like, "he's a jerk" or "he's inconsiderate." And that may be true, but probably not everyone is thinking about that person incessantly, being angry at night trying to figure out ways to avoid them or get back at them. Thus, if not every person is having the same experience as us, then the answer might be: "It's us." Maybe it's us who needs to look inside and has to change. A lot of this book is about ownership, a personal sense of responsibility for our choices, feelings and thoughts.

Why would we want to take ownership?

1. We can't change other people anyway no matter how hard we try or want to. So, from a practical and energy standpoint, changing ourselves makes a lot of sense.

2. Change is not torture. It's a gift to our own selves, a signal to look deeper inside.

3. When we change due to the lessons others provide for us, we feel more connected to them and to the world.

4. Releasing old patterns removes toxic energy and improves our health.

5. Once we learn a particular lesson from a situation, we are less likely to repeat the mental/emotional pattern we experience in it. We can move on from it and begin to have *new* experiences *in the same situation.*

CAVEAT: Having practiced looking inward for things about myself to change for years now, I know that if the same situation appears again and again, it means I haven't learned the lesson!

The White Coat Supremacy

One day, when I was a medical student working in the pediatric ward, one of the higher-up residents stopped me and told me that it would be better if I didn't wear my white lab coat. When I asked her why, she explained that children are scared of the white coat, because when they see it, it means bad things (like pills and shots) are going to happen. As a result, pediatric patients would be less inclined to be open and receptive if I wore it. Since that day, I decided that wearing the white coat was something I would try to avoid, even with adults. It's already intimidating enough to be sitting in a doctor's office with a medical problem, let alone having someone come in who visually has more power than you, or even worse yet, reminds you of "bad things" from your childhood. I have noticed that some doctors don't really seem to care whether or not they are well received; rather they rely on the statistics, facts and innate authority they have as diploma-carrying doctors. Somewhat jokingly, I call these types of doctors, "The White Coats."

I know as soon as hardline White Coat-ers read this book, they will dismiss blocked energy being a potential cause of disease because there are no Western style double-blind studies to support it. This is understandable because of how we were trained in school, where evidence was king. Don't get me wrong though. I am a big believer in evidence and the scientific method. Where I stand now, my stepwise approach to Western medicine is this:

1. If a Western treatment works above 90%, then go for it! You have a cure! Go do it. As I mentioned earlier, not all diseases are caused by problems in more than one House. If you have a disease that is curable in over 90% of cases, then by all means, please do it. (You will still have to deal with the underlying causes, but at least you'll be out of immediate danger.)

2. If the cure rate is below 25% or there is no cure, then we either need to do something completely different or add to the current Western treatment.

3. If you see the words, "Idiopathic" or "Essential" or "Autoimmune" in the scientific name, you can rest assured we have no *real* clue how to truly heal the condition. Think about it: When we, the White Coats, don't know how or why a disease comes about, why would you agree to the proposed solution? As a patient, I wouldn't agree, at least not that treatment on its own. If I told you that I couldn't do better than a 50% chance to help you (and sometimes much less than that) why on Earth would you accept that? Because you believe that you don't have an alternative? Well, there is an alternative, and that is usually to *add* to the current treatment. In this book, I'm offering you a way to look at things differently, a way in which you have control and responsibility. Yes, I certainly will agree with you, it *is* much easier to just "do what the doctor says."

4. People are often faced with a decision to either do a minimally effective treatment or do nothing. In Western literature, researchers sometimes trumpet "a statistically significant three months improvement in survival in a randomized trial" as if it were a life-altering achievement (like in pancreatic cancer or lung

cancer.) Some of this is due to the fact that in many diseases, we are desperate for a positive result, and some of this is due to the fact that pharmaceutical companies have spent millions on developing the drug, and they need to be able to make their money back. If I were a patient facing this decision, I would probably think, "Come on, really? You want me to take a treatment that potentially gives me MORE side effects and suffering AND has only a 50% chance of extending my life an average of THREE more months? Really?" Let me be clear though. I am not saying doing a minimally effective therapy is wrong. I'm saying it's worth it to consider a *different way of thinking*. Why consider a different way? Let someone much smarter than me tell you what he thinks:

"Insanity: doing the same thing over and over again and expecting a different result."

-Albert Einstein

This quote may be directed more at entrenched doctors, who, by staying "by the book" in their field, may miss some key information, whether in nontraditional research, or even supplied by his/her patients. If these practitioners' psyches were more flexible, perhaps they would be open to alternative ways of improving overall health, and by doing so, could aid in the process of empowering their patients to facilitate their own healing.

I can't tell you how many times I have heard from patients about astonishing, complementary treatments they have discovered on their own. The truth is, many times patients won't even mention complementary treatments if they feel their doctor isn't open to them. So, what happens (more often than not) is that these amazing "discoveries" are left to researchers, not practitioners. Thankfully, I had some great role models (and patients!) in my life who taught me to listen and then do my own investigation to see if that new knowledge is A.: True, and if true then B.: incorporate into my own knowledge base.

"Listening is being able to be changed by the other person."
-Alan Alda,
actor, director, screenwriter, author

One of my greatest driving forces growing up was my mother, who continually pushed me to achieve more. I can remember a time when I scored a 99% on a test and was asked by my mom, "Why did you miss this last one?" when I got home. (Google "Tiger Mom" for more details on this type of Asian mom!) While this was oftentimes tough emotionally growing up, as an adult I can see that it galvanized in me a deeply imprinted desire to know and learn as much as possible, not to "rest on my laurels." Also because of my mom, I am always ready to adapt, to be really open to a new way of doing things, even if inside I get "puffed up" by hearing some critical comments. So, when I ask you as the reader to consider accepting responsibility and asking to make big changes in your health and awareness, I do it with personal experience of how that might feel: anxiety-filled and very hard to accept.

Another person who was crucial to the way I approach knowledge was Dr. Juillard. He had a straightforward and modest saying that rings in my ears to this very day (especially when I am feeling overly impressed with myself):

"There is always room for improvement."

Dr. Juillard would say this to residents and patients alike when he himself was presented with a new way of looking at a disease. It was a wonderful sign of his humility and also a strong indication of his mastery of patient care. Even after forty years of clinical practice, he never seemed offended by a suggestion from someone who had less experience than he, because he knew that he might just learn something new.

You may feel that I am beating you over the head with this concept, but here it is again: *Take ownership of your health!* (I will say it many more times before this book is done.)

Oftentimes, patients try to rationalize to me a passive approach to health. They may refer to it as "Trusting the doctor" or may bring up the old adage "Doctor knows best." This attitude was more widely held with older generations and, lamentably, still prevails in certain parts of the U.S. and abroad. However, in this day and age, with shorter windows for doctors to see patients, ever-expanding ways in which to attack a disease, and much easier access to information, this passive attitude towards health is selling ourselves way short (and in some cases can be dangerous). Many doctors still believe that nutrition plays no role in recovery, and I see it much too often unfortunately in cancer care. Even though there is ample research (as well as common sense!) supporting increased vegetable and fruit intake, this is still not widely recommended. If you do a brief Internet search (or read further in this book) you'll see there is a lot we are learning with regards to nutrition.

Takeaway: *Even if a Western medicine treatment has an 80-90% success rate, you STILL need to be the captain of your own wellness ship.*

It is not rare that a patient might not want to do a particular treatment but feels pressured into doing it. Sometimes the patient feels forced into a certain type of treatment, either by the doctor or by the patient's family. As I said earlier, no matter what a doctor says, *you are truly the one responsible and the one "in charge."* A doctor cannot prescribe any treatment without your consent. That is what a consent form is for, to ensure that you, the patient are voluntarily signing on to a treatment. I, personally, even with a consent form signed, never start a treatment without the patient being fully on board mentally and emotionally. Why? Because as Dr. Juillard said:

"We cannot treat you without you."

Stop Blaming the Conspiracy

When I hear people talk about the "conspiratorial" effort by the medical industry to suppress the cure for cancer, I sort of just shake my head. They make it sound like there's a systematic, resolute effort to prevent "the truth" from coming out. Some of my conspiracy-theorist friends even go as far as to state that *all* doctors "are in it just to make money." Yes, medicine is a business. Part of having a business is making money, and some doctors go beyond the bounds of ethics and law, and then the law prosecutes them when they are eventually discovered to be performing unethical procedures. I personally know hundreds of doctors and the unscrupulous are the minority of doctors. Rather than focusing on making gobs of money, most doctors struggle with huge loans, burnout, not spending enough time with their families, and drowning under the paperwork of the healthcare insurance industry. Most of the doctors I have met and worked with are compassionate, caring people who are doing their best in this conflicting era of limited resources. Believing in some massive, institutionalized cover-up, to me, is a waste of energy that detracts from actually finding out what YOU need to do to be healthy.

Why hasn't cancer been cured? The truth is, we aren't smart enough yet. We just don't know how to cure some cancers at a high rate. It's as simple as that.

Cancer is such a complex disease, with multiple things going wrong in multiple places (often 60-100 malfunctions and mutations in each tumor) that a "magic bullet," in the form of a pill, still couldn't cure anything on its own. It is perplexing and frustrating. Even when we try a new drug and it has a dramatic killing effect, the remaining cancer cells mutate and defiantly get around the drug, making the cancer even stronger because it has become more resistant. The drug has killed only the weaker cells and the strong survive.

The fact is that with some of the most-known cancers (i.e., pancreatic, brain, lung) the cure rates are appalling, only 10-15% in many cases. This disturbing truth, often shattering for the patient, is also tormenting for the doctor. There are some remarkable advances happening research-wise, especially using the body's own immune system (virus and vaccine therapies to name two) to fight cancer, but these findings are still early in development.

I once had a patient with an incurable brain cancer. He had two adorable kids. When he brought his children into the clinic, my heart just sank. Not only was he exactly my age at the time, 35, but I knew that he wouldn't live to see his kids' next five years. I wanted so much to say to him, "We can cure you," to tell his kids, "We can cure your daddy." But that would have been a lie. With the treatments that I had knowledge of, it was a near certainty that he would die. As doctors, it's a tragic and humbling process to prescribe a treatment that only works 10-15% of the time.

One thing I have learned in my life and in my practice, especially in the past few years, is that our thoughts create much of our reality. Even in the science of medicine, with its pragmatic approach and sometimes strict dogma, what we believe to be true (for doctor and patient alike) often becomes our reality. This can have a significant effect on overall health and healing.

As human beings, we get our attitudes, beliefs and "truths" from the powerful messages in society, and those notions and ideas become ingrained within us, even if they are inaccurate, incorrect, or no longer apply. Forty years ago, "cancer" was a death sentence. The cure rate overall now is above 70% for all stages of cancer, and over 85% for early stages, including the most common like breast and prostate cancer. Still, friends on the street will have the impression that it's uniformly fatal. I will correct them, and a surprised look will cross their face, even sometimes dismissing what I have said. Even with professionals, the concept that a "malignant brain tumor is fatal" is deeply rooted in our collective medical consciousness. This belief that such a formidable disease cannot be altered, forms an acceptance of the status quo. "That's just the way it is," we tell ourselves, because so far, no one has seen any contrary results. Living in this mindset, we begin to buy into the perception, "Who are we to believe that we can do better?" This grim mentality is called "therapeutic nihilism."

Nihilism is the contention that what we are doing is worthless or totally useless. Turning it back to the concept of ownership, if we as doctors accept that there is "nothing that can be done," it takes the pressure off of us to find something new. It relieves us of the responsibility to find another way. It keeps our egos undamaged and allows us to feel somewhat less guilty in our notion that we tried all that is available to us.

I really feel that it takes great courage to admit that we don't know it all. Doctors are not omniscient. We are mere mortals like everyone else and so much is unknown to us. Once we can accept and choose to live *with the discomfort of not knowing*, then we can begin to look for alternative sources of inspiration and possibility. It takes a certain fearlessness to accept that we have so much more to learn. Even the best, bravest and most open-minded doctors face untold challenges in trying to modify the system. Fears of malpractice, litigation and retribution are just a scratching of the surface.

My point in telling you this background is to let you see what is *really* going on behind the scenes. When you hear someone blaming the medical establishment in a sweeping, generalized way, they may be operating either from a place of ignorance or a place of pain from a bad experience, but certainly not from reality. This unhelpful perspective as a patient is as rigid a stance as is the position of the doctor who chooses to see no new options.

A Cancer Success Story

A type of cancer called lymphoma is a great example of this willingness to try something different, over and over. In the last sixty years cure rates for lymphoma have gone from 50% in the 1960s eventually to the present day statistic of 90%. To achieve this, it has taken a combination of four to five different chemotherapeutic drugs at different intensities and dosages (sometimes coupled with radiation) just to get to this level of remarkable progress. That's forty years of testing and retesting, with successes and failure along the way. Without the perseverance and courage to try new things, this 40% increase in survival would never have been possible and thousands of human beings would have died in the meantime.

> *"Ever tried. Ever failed. No matter. Try again. Fail again. Fail better."*
>
> - Samuel Beckett,
> from *Worstward Ho*[ii]

Why Bother Learning This Stuff?

Why are you reading this book? I can only assume that it is because you are making the effort to empower yourself with knowledge and insight. Well, I have some good news!

Although it seems like there's always new discoveries to keep up with, it is really not this ever-changing, always growing information that has the most potent effect on your health. It is effort and persistence that are the keys to being healthier. Simply making the effort, and never giving up, will lead you to success with your health. How awesome is that?

I can appreciate how bewildering it seems to be living in a time where the old saying, "An apple a day keeps the doctor away" has morphed into "An organic, locally-grown, pesticide-free apple a day (plus kale, broccoli and Brussels sprouts) can improve your immune surveillance." Fortunately, because of this refined and increasing knowledge, we are living longer than ever before.

I was born in 1974. That year, U.S. life expectancy was 74 years old. Now it is 79. In forty years, the average life expectancy has increased by *five* years. This may seem insignificant, but to put this number into perspective, in scientific studies an increase of six *months* in life expectancy due to a treatment is considered compelling.

How did it happen that we managed to extend American's lives by five years? It came about because people started to learn which foods, activities, and lifestyles were good for them and which were not. Additionally, there have been significant advances in medical care of the main killers, especially for heart disease, stroke, and cancer. This is another reminder that a combination of the best of Western medicine and the best of holistic knowledge is the key.

Okay, so we are living longer, and I am sure you know many people who have lived way beyond this average age of 79. The more important question to me actually is: How is our quality of life in those extra years? Stated in another way, what does it matter if we live five more years, if in those years we are riddled with pain and suffering?

Another reason why I wrote this book was because in 1974, a lot of the knowledge of personal health was unknown or at least, not readily available to the public. Now, with the explosion of the information age, we can learn the things to make those years of expanded life expectancy as joyful and healthy as possible. A lot of them are in this book. The great news is that we will probably learn to live even longer! Here's something to shoot for: The average Japanese life expectancy is 84, five years longer than in the United States! Why, might you ask? Most researchers point to their diet, which is full of antioxidants and maybe more importantly, 60-80% lower in calories.[iii]

Be Aware When You Read Stuff on the Internet

The following scenario has happened to me on too many occasions and it is worth sharing. A friend diagnosed with cancer comes to me (unaware that I am in the field of cancer treatment) and proclaims, "You need to check out this website. I read the articles and the treatments and I cured myself! Forget those doctors!"

"You don't feel the Western treatment worked?" I ask.

"No," the friend replies. "I had to do it all myself."

After probing further, I find out what the real story is and it usually takes two forms.

The first scenario is that they actually have received the full Western treatment (most of the time this means surgery, radiation and/or chemotherapy) but are unhappy with the way they were treated or they feel like the side effects weren't acceptable. Often, they feel that their doctor didn't take the time to listen to them or they experienced a side effect that they felt shouldn't have happened. So, they feel frustrated, angry and even abandoned. And because of this, they throw the baby out with the bathwater, so to speak, and dismiss or denounce even the parts of treatment that may have been beneficial. They simply generalize their overall experience into an emotional sound bite, leaving those who are listening to believe that the treatment didn't work.

The second scenario I often find with people who tout their self-cure is that their diagnosis oftentimes *isn't even cancer*. Many times, after some fact checking, I see their diagnosis is actually listed as a "tumor" which is merely a general term for some kind of growth. The word "tumor" is not interchangeable with "cancer." It is important to note that the word "tumor" does not indicate if it is benign or malignant. As a general rule, benign tumors (by definition) do not have the ability to kill you. Malignant ones do and only malignant tumors are truly "cancer."

Now don't get me wrong: it can be very difficult not to be influenced by a passionate testimonial, especially by someone who is close to you. My point is that we need to ask more questions and probe deeper this person's claims of healing by diet or herbs alone. It is absolutely imperative that we have the full information when we determine how much value to give to those stories.

Sometimes, those stories come from our own lives. I have had patients who were so scared of a potential treatment because of the horror they remember from the past, whether as a child or even more recently. Many times, I have heard, "radiation burned my uncle's neck, that's why he died," or "they gave him radiation to his brain, he lost his hair and it killed him." The emotional trauma of a loved one dying often makes us ascribe blame to relieve ourselves, at least partly, from feeling the sadness and helplessness that can overcome us. Once I get more facts, I can often redirect people into what actually was going on. For the two test cases above, radiation causes burns often during treatment (called radiation dermatitis) and especially in head and neck cancers, those burns can be very dramatic. They do heal, but oftentimes the cancers are advanced and that is what caused the death. In the second case, radiation is given to the brain when there are brain metastases, and even with treatment the average survival is low, averaging less than a year. It is very understandable to have these misunderstandings but it becomes even more tragic when patients refuse a potentially curative treatment because of inaccurate associations.

There's "Science" ... And Then There's Science.

As medical doctors, we are inundated throughout our careers and lives with study after study looking at a slew of different scientific questions. We become experts at reading these studies, determining why one study may be more valid through its experimental design or why it may be more consequential due to its more "statistically significant" results than previous studies on the subject. It is an essential critical thinking skill to be able to determine a study's inherent significance and is something quality medical doctors do not take lightly. This ability allows us to be gatekeepers to new therapies, which is an enormous responsibility. We are taught in medical school to prioritize "evidence-based" treatments. To be able to really understand in a rational, intelligent, and fine-tuned way if a new treatment is actually worth doing is of paramount importance for our patients.

There is a downside, however, to this evidence-based critical analysis, and it usually takes two forms. Firstly, after years and years of looking at studies, we stop asking, "Was this study even worth doing?" Instead, we tend to focus on whether the study was well done or not.

Sometimes, I see studies that waste millions of dollars and [even more importantly] valuable time, to answer questions that have already been well covered in the past. These redundant reports are more about a researcher getting a paper published by a leading journal rather than actually contributing to worthwhile and potentially life-changing exploration. It's no longer a surprise to me to see some "new" study that duplicates one done over twenty years ago, just with different authors!

The second thing that often happens from academic study of experiments is that we as doctors get disconnected with what we really are doing in the clinic. Too frequently, we like to believe that we *only* use methods derived from scientific studies. When we get an inspiration to try something new, we may stop ourselves and first ask, "Is there data to support this?" Oftentimes, we refrain from considering a new way because there is little data.

Having an inspiration and no data to support it means we are left in the unknown, exposed to the fear of lawsuits that may arise should something go wrong or worse yet, harming the patient we are trying to help. Moreover, I have personally felt disheartened when offering the same "tried and true" treatments that *do not cure the disease,* simply because that is the standard of care. (The standard of care means what is generally accepted as "best practice" or what has been practiced for many years.) In advanced stage lung cancer for example, the *improvement* in survival with combined chemotherapy, radiation and biologic therapy over best supportive care (meaning keeping the person comfortable without any radical treatments) is still measured in months not years. This is with best efforts and multimillion dollars in research. Insurance companies also provide a barrier to trying new things as they only approve treatments that have been thoroughly validated. Some patients are able to fight through the bureaucracy to get something new, but for the most part the only way a patient gets an experimental therapy is through a clinical trial funded by the pharmaceutical company that makes the therapy or if the clinical trial is funded by an outside source such as the National Institutes of Health.

Let me be clear though, what I am saying is not to abandon the current treatment for any cancer, but to be open to new ways of doing things, oftentimes brought by the patients themselves. Even if we cannot advocate for these new ideas, either for ethical reasons or legal reasons, we must not shut down the patient's initiative to survive and follow their instincts.

Also, the *reality* is that some of the biggest breakthroughs in science have been discovered *not* through "rigorous experimental design" (double-blind studies testing one treatment against another) but rather good old-fashioned trial-and-error (let's try it and see if it works) or even by accident. Penicillin was famously discovered by accident when Sir Alexander Fleming, a Scottish researcher, returned from vacation to find mold on an accidentally contaminated staphylococcus culture plate. Smallpox, a killer of untold millions for centuries, was stopped by a word of mouth story that a farmer and his family were immune to smallpox due to a cow virus they had been infected with. Edward Jenner, an English physician, testing out this story, found that the cow virus certainly did prevent the smallpox infection from occurring. This eventually led to the vaccination movement and saved millions of lives from infection and death due to smallpox.

In short, sometimes ingenuity comes from unlikely sources and we must be open to the possibility!

In much the same way as a doctor must be open, as an individual looking to heal any disease, we must be prepared to step away from simply accepting "what has been done" into something new. What is necessary now for your best health and an empowered sense of wellness is a fresh trust in a new way of doing things. By "trying out and seeing" a new way, you might get to *feel* the results within you. Sometimes well-intentioned friends can suggest the same thing three or four times and we on the receiving end of the suggestion just do not have the open-mindedness to even consider it. I have had this experience myself, many times, probably due to being stubborn, most memorably with the habit of eating dairy. I was told by multiple people, "Maybe your stomach issues are because of milk and cheese?" I ignored it for years because of my love of adding cheese to everything. Instead of stopping dairy, I started adding more and more lactose digestion pills, trying to keep up with my dairy habit, getting more and more symptoms, (stomach pain, rashes, lots of mucus, nosebleeds) with each passing month. (You can read the resolution to the story later in the book.)

The reason I tell this story is to let you know, I know how hard it is to change a habit, and also how hard it is to try a new way. As human beings, we are all afraid [to some degree] of the unknown. That is why many of us remain in familiar but unsuccessful patterns of health and wellness rather than challenging our comfort zones for something possibly better out in those uncharted waters. I see a lot of people go through terrible angst before starting a different kind of treatment because of the foreign landscape that lies beyond the decision to try. I expect no different a reaction from anyone trying to change something deeply ingrained. What may be helpful to you when considering trying out something I suggest in this book is to ask yourself these four questions:

1. **Is the way I am doing things working?** If the answer is yes, then keep doing it. But if the answer is "No, things are not working," then you have to ask yourself the second question:

2. **Am I *ready* to try something different?** Being "ready" means, are you willing to give up the way you are doing things, and mentally try something new, even before hearing the new way. And once you have heard the new way, then you are willing to try it. This is being "ready."

3. **In your intuitional, or gut feeling, does the new way feel right for you?** This initial feeling, experienced usually with an inner sense of calmness, is your guide to change.

4. **Are you willing to give the new way an honest trial period?** (Even if you do not see results immediately?)

Question three is a difficult one. So often, most patients are terrified, so scared in fact that it's very difficult to get them to stop worrying and really figure out what feels right on a gut level. It is hard for any of us to consider what feels right when we are frightened. (We will look at ways in the Spiritual House to try and help you hear that voice, the main way being meditation.) What I try to do is to help take the pressure off my patients by encouraging them to give it a try. I tell them, "If you find it's not working for you, you just stop."

Question number four has been shown to be very hard to do as well. In a study called the PURE study of 153,996 people who have had a heart attack or stroke, 25% of subjects made no changes to their eating, exercise or smoking habits. Only 4.3% of people were able to change all three to any significant degree.[iv] This shows us how hard it can be to change even if our life is clearly on the line. Sometimes we have to go a few weeks or even a few months to see if something induces a change in us that we can actually point at and say, "Yes, this actually worked!" In my experience, that new way may not even be the "final" answer but can often be a bridge to something more permanent.

A trial period is a great idea because not *every* way works for *every*body: A particular way or method of doing things may or may not work for you. Sometimes the subconscious makes us believe, "If we start this, we'll have to do it forever." That's not true. If it's not working, you stop. Simple. What we are looking for is a habit of trying new things. Sometimes it takes a few attempts at new things before one of them is the right fit. Yes, family members or friends who were initially excited at your trying something new may be disappointed, but we are not talking about going back to the old ways. We are talking about moving forward and trying something *else* if the first way doesn't work for you. I have often recommended a new approach to people and months later, have reconnected with them to find that they had stopped what I suggested and actually found something else that gave them the result they were looking for, and were grateful, as one person said, to have had "their motor kick-started!"

And remember: When it comes to your personal health and wellness, you are the captain of your own ship. You cannot be coerced into any treatment against your will. And you certainly can't be forced to continue something that doesn't feel right and/or isn't working. The choices are yours to make!

The Autoimmune Issue

Our human bodies have an exquisitely sensitive monitoring system for detecting invaders in the body. This is called *immune surveillance.* It is how the body defends itself against attacks from bacteria, viruses and other pathogens that may enter from what we eat, drink, breathe or even through our skin. Oftentimes though, the immune system can overreact or become hypersensitive to things that actually are not harmful to it, interpreting something harmless as being unsafe.

When the immune system believes another part of the body is abnormal, it attacks it. If the immune system is miscalibrated, our bodies can inappropriately start to attack nerves, organs, pretty much anything in the body. This state is what western medicine calls an *autoimmune disease*. If what is being attacked is essential to the survival of your body, it becomes an enormous problem. I'm sure you can imagine how dangerous this can be. Unfortunately, assigning a label, e.g. the word "autoimmune," to the problem doesn't mean that it offers a solution.

Oftentimes I hear people say, "I'm just relieved that now I know what it is." As human beings, there is often great comfort in putting a name to something because not being able to define what is wrong with us causes profound anxiety and fear. So, from a patient's perspective, suffering may be diminished simply by knowing that they have something that someone else, especially a professional, has heard of before, because now they are not alone. This sense of comfort is no small thing. However, from my perspective as a healer, it doesn't really offer any concrete help beyond a starting point.

For example, let's take the disease called ITP. It stands for Idiopathic Thrombocytopenic Purpura. Let's break down this intimidating name:

Idiopathic - "arising spontaneously or from an unknown cause."

Thrombocytopenic – low platelet count.

Purpura - purple-colored spots on the skin.

So, if we translate the name, based on the above breakdown, it simply means: "I don't know why, but you have a low platelet count and purple spots on your skin." The name tells us right away that the scientific community has little to no understanding of how ITP develops! It simply describes what is seen in the body.

Do you get my point? To me, it doesn't matter what the name is if doctors don't know how to treat it! Much more can and should be done.

As a doctor, it is fascinating to me that part of the definition of "idiopathic" means "arising spontaneously." Let's be quite clear, shall we? No disease ever "arises spontaneously." EVER. Nothing *just happens.* Everything in the body has a reason for being the way that it is.

If you have a disease that doesn't currently have an explanation as to why it occurred, it doesn't mean that an explanation doesn't exist. It may take time, trial and error to find an explanation and a treatment but one almost always exists. It may sound encouraging and at the same time daunting, but sometimes that is the point of life, isn't it? What one learns on the journey is the reason one starts the journey in the first place. There have been many times in my life where I have asked myself, "Why!?" and felt the dread of the unknown, worrying how things were going to turn out because I could not see a clear endpoint. By going forward step-by-step through many of these experiences and continuing to be persistent, I have built a muscle in me, a strength that comes only through experience, a knowing that I am better off for going through it. I know if you look back at your life and remember times like these, you have always made it through and been better for it, at least on the inside of your being and more likely on the outside as well. Of all of the people whom I have met that have taken this journey into the unknown for their own healing, very few regret it.

> *"When you walk to the edge of all the light you have and take that first step into the darkness of the unknown, you must believe that one of two things will happen. There will be something solid for you to stand upon or you will be taught how to fly."*
>
> - Patrick Overton, *The Leaning Tree*[v]

Your Body's Set Point for Health

Our bodies, vigilant in their desire to protect and serve our best interests of health and wellness, constantly screen our cells to make sure that they are normal. This process is called immunoediting[vi]. Our bodies are equipped with the amazing mechanism of removing defective cells by sending a signal to cause these defective cells to basically self-destruct. The fact that the correct signal is being sent thousands of times a day to the appropriate cells is a miracle in itself! This astonishing process is called *apoptosis.*

One way to look at the problem of cancer is to see it as a profound *loss* of the body's natural ability to find these offending cells and remove them. Ideally, the body should respond to something that isn't supposed to be there, but in many cancer cases, there is literally no reaction to the life threatening mutant cells. For a system (the human body) that is a continuous miracle in action with millions of signaling communications and adjustments occurring every second, does it not seem strange and disturbing that the body does not react aggressively to something so profoundly wrong as cancer? Why is this?

Although much of this immunity research is still in its infancy, I have come to understand and explain it this way: The cells of our bodies are continuously regenerating themselves, day after day, year after year. In spite of debilitating environmental pressures, like stress, pollution, exposure to toxins like cigarettes and alcohol, our amazing body keeps producing new and functional cells to keep our body alive and working, taking defective cells out of circulation.

However, the accumulation of harmful stressors on the body eventually takes its toll, and the cells that are remaining in circulation become less and less healthy. Over time, the body is forced to lower its standard for what constitutes a healthy cell. If the body didn't do this, then too large a percentage of cells would be labeled defective and have to be destroyed, which inevitably would kill the body. The body rightly prioritizes *survival over perfection.* But this lowering of standards is a dangerous practice because at some point, the body will allow a cell to "pass security" when the cell should have been destroyed. At this point, a cancer cell can form and escape the body's surveillance system, *because it is so close to what a "normal cell" looks like that the body cannot tell the difference.*

Immune research is also demonstrating that once a cancer cell has taken root and started to grow, it produces chemicals that inhibit immune pathways (the two most studied are called PD-1[vii] and CTLA-4[viii] but there are many) that are critical "checkpoints" to recognizing cancer cells. In a sense, cancer makes these "security guards" fall asleep, so cancer can grow and thrive without being seen. This is evidenced by some emerging studies that show a nonexistent immune response and/or low antibody levels in certain (but not all) cancers. Even when powerful treatments such as chemotherapies, radiation and biologic targeted drugs are used, we find that the cancers can often recur, most likely due to this combined effect of the lowering of the immune surveillance and also the tricky methods of the cancer itself to hijack the immune system and make sure it's not seen.

Much of the current research is being spent on developing new drugs to unblock these immune checkpoints like PD-1 and CTLA-4. There are exciting breakthroughs almost every few months and of course this work is much needed for those who develop cancer. My goal in this book is to focus on what we can do that is within our personal control, *before* cancer develops. Even though life takes its toll on our bodies, we still have an ability to help our immune system, not just by stopping unhealthy habits, but also by *adding* and integrating fun and healthy habits in our lives, like the ones to be presented in upcoming chapters.

Why Choosing to Make Changes is Important

When I first counsel people looking to make life changes, I can often sense the anxiety, fear, and dejectedness that comes along with even *hearing* about proposed alterations. I totally understand this and can relate. It's a daunting thing to change something, especially when it is so ingrained in our lives. This is particularly true when it comes to diet.

Eating is an extremely emotional thing. Food means love in many cultures and it is one of the only ways some cultures express care and concern. I can still clearly remember that moment when I first told my mom that I was stopping eating beef and pork. My mom has always shown her love through the foods she prepares for us. I knew it might be a tough conversation so I approached it gently.

"Mom, maybe when I come up to visit, can we have mostly fish and tofu instead of beef?"

"You don't like my cooking?" she immediately replied.

"No, that is not it. I love your cooking."

"Why don't you like my cooking anymore?"

"Mom ..."

To her, on a deep level it felt like I was disowning our traditions, even though I was looking out for my health and indirectly my parents as well. For the next few trips home, she would stubbornly still make the same dishes and put them out in front of me.

"Eat it. It's good!"

Of course, I am not twelve years old anymore (although mothers have a way of making that fact irrelevant). I didn't fight, even though I was a little frustrated. I just ate around the red meat. It was challenging for a few visits home, but eventually she realized I had made up my mind to change. Eventually she realized that my personal dietary changes were not an affront to her. She adapted by cooking dishes that fit both my dad and me. In the end, taking that risk for my health and well-being turned out even better than I expected. She even started to cook brown rice instead of white rice when I came up to visit, much to the chagrin of my father! (My dad: "You only cook what he wants!")

In order to help combat the problematic but understandable "separation anxiety" that my patients feel in detaching from familiar but unhealthy habits, I try to provide some awareness. I ask them, "How bad are the problems you're having right now? Are they affecting your quality of life to the point that you need to change?" That's a question I ask you now as well: Are you ready to change?

I have a lot of experience in helping people change, and I have found time and again that people *will* change, but only when they have suffered enough and can't tolerate the status quo any longer.

If we step back for a moment and take a larger perspective, perhaps we can recognize that every experience we have in life is an opportunity to learn and to grow. Looking at it this way, maybe the issues that are coming up time and again, provoking a need for change, are meant for our highest good. Maybe the lessons to be learned here, even in the face of adversity, are meant as an opportunity to learn lessons to bring you closer to the real You.

A monk once told me, "First God taps you, then He pokes you, then He kicks you, then …well then… He stops talking and lets the world teach you." Even if you don't believe in God, you will find that life will continue to challenge you with the same conditions over and over again until you learn the lesson the situation is trying to teach you.

There is, of course, a more elegant way to change, and a way that is less painful. I cite it as "The Way of Wisdom."

Take it from me, for many years I didn't choose wisdom either! There have been and will continue to be times in our lives when we just don't want to listen. That being said, wouldn't you rather have it be that *you* choose the time to change, rather than the world shoving it right in your face? In the case of health, this rude awakening by the world could mean getting a disease you never believed could happen or having a recurrence of a disease that you thought was cured. When we decide to make change rather than having change thrust upon us, we empower ourselves for the greatest opportunity to transform our lives for the better. In the short term it may feel painful, but in the long term that is rarely the case.

Goal Setting

As students coming up through our educational system, we are taught from a very early age that we have to pass a test in order to graduate and go forward. This seems like a great way to assess ourselves after finishing school: Give ourselves tests, or goals to shoot for. This seems like a smart and commonsense approach to achieve things, but what I have witnessed repeatedly is that people love to set extraordinarily high, nearly-impossible-to-meet goals. They then go after them with unsustainable fervor and un-reasonable expectations. Whether it is a radical new diet, a "revolutionary" workout regimen, or the good old standby, the New Year's resolution, people often dive in blindly and anticipate miracles, sometimes achieving a short-lived thirty-pound weight loss only to balloon when a period of stress causes them to overeat again. In short, overly idealistic goal setting creates an unhealthy, often nerve-racking pressure to achieve something that even if reached, cannot be sustained.

Goal setting can become not just idealistic but also competitive. I grew up in an extremely competitive environment, where everything became a rivalry of sorts. I competed against everyone for everything: grades, sports and even food eating. At the dinner table, my brother and I were consistently challenging each other to receive my mother's pleased exhortations such as, "Wow, you drank the whole half gallon of milk today!" In my family, we even had a running tally for years of who won the most Ping-Pong games between my dad, my brother and myself. (Full disclosure: I did the tallying!)

Competitive goal setting works pretty well for sports and school, which are controlled environments, in which outcome is measured through numbers. What about in real life? Not so good. It's not a wise idea to compete in conversations, vie for victory while driving in traffic, or create a contest out of health. Especially with social media, it can be dangerous to our self-esteem when we see someone we admire (or even more provoking, someone we are jealous of) lose a lot of weight in a short period of time, which puts pressure on us to do the same. The tunnel vision of social media can make it seem as if weight loss was the only endpoint for health and happiness!

When we set up expectations about our health, we often make assumptions about our ability to control all aspects of our wellness. We get lulled into believing that reaching our "goal" is just a matter of sheer willpower and hard work. We don't take into account the internal and external factors that can affect the possible outcome. The first and most damaging of these assumptions is that a goal is something that once reached, is the end of the journey.

Take, for instance, dieting. How many "diets" have you gone on over the years? How many times have you set a seemingly reasonable expectation for yourself? How many times have you reached your benchmark? How many times have you sustained your goal once you have achieved it? (Seriously, take a minute and write down how many diets you have attempted, completed and maintained.)

Even with goals that seem sensible, there are many factors besides willpower that determine if we fall short, are forced to quit, or slide back once we "arrive" at our destination. Looking just at weight loss, factors such as genetics, preexisting conditions, hormone imbalances, neural circuitry, hyperpalatable foods (those made cheaply and great tasting), addiction, finances and misinformation are all a part of the success/failure equation. In many ways, the deck is already stacked against us.

Many of life's great accomplishments are part of a process that always changes, fluctuates, and has no real ending. Being a good father, mother, sister, brother, son, daughter, lover, teacher, friend; these things have no specific endpoint. They are ongoing. They require sustained effort and perpetual care. How can they be measured in fixed goals or prospects set in stone? When we approach them as things to check off our bucket list, we are setting ourselves up for demoralizing outcomes and near certain failure.

So, what should we do? Well, I have a *truly radical* idea:

Don't set goals when it comes to health.

"What are you saying, Dr. Roy? This goes against everything I've been taught."

Please. Hear me out.

There is a concept in Japan called *kaizen*, which is defined as "continuous daily improvement." Basically, what this means is that every day, try to be a little bit better than the day before. This is how *real change* happens, lasting change. And this is something that we all want, isn't it? Ironically, if you think about it, "continuous daily improvement" *is* a goal, an achievable and humble one at that. It may not be sexy or "fit for a Facebook post" but it's sustainable and achievable!

Habits Are Us

The title of this section is in honor of my friend Dr. Jim Keefe, who has a class he gives for people who are looking to change habits, whether it's overeating, smoking or lack of exercise. (His talk is available on YouTube if you want to check it out!) I don't want to "steal his thunder" but I will say that I do agree with two of his main points: The only real internal thing you need to have in order to change a bad habit is willpower. The second thing that I agree with: if you can afford it, a coach is helpful to keep you on track.

The research on habit formation is helpful to know, as it can help us form new good habits. There are five main points:

1. Small repeatable changes are proven to stick.[ix] You have to choose something that you can "kaizen" every day. For example, making a small dietary change rather than a wholesale lifestyle change, e.g. committing to eating one carrot everyday rather than becoming a vegetarian. Also, trying to add variety has been shown to be not as effective as picking one thing and repeating it.

2. It takes approximately 10 weeks to reach a plateau where the new behavior becomes automatic.[x] This means you have to commit to doing it every day for ten weeks before you will feel "weird" that you did *not* do the behavior. This makes it more understandable why you want to pick something easy to do.

3. Conquering one small change will increase your self-esteem and also your motivation to make bigger changes. Think of habit formation as a muscle: You've got to start with a smaller weight before moving to the heavier ones. Conversely, failing at a new behavior will make it less likely you'll try again.

4. You have to *add* a new behavior, not just take one away. Your mind cannot make a habit of *not* doing something.

5. Contextual cueing: Set up your new behavior for success by linking it to something you already are habitually doing. For example, if you want to add a short walk to your day, pair it with your breakfast. After you eat breakfast, that's when you go for a short walk. (Of course, this example is schedule dependent.) The context of breakfast will *cue* your mind to know, "Hey, we are going for a walk after this."

Getting Unstuck

Are you feeling some anxiety? It's hard to get started, right? So, how do we get going after so long of NOT going?

Imagine that you are on a boat sitting in the port. Off in the distance, you see an island. It is quite a distance away but there is something about it that is intriguing to you, something that MIGHT be promising. "I wonder what that island is like," you first think to yourself. But quickly, your thoughts race to those of concern: "What if I don't like that island? What if it's not as good as this port? What if it's a waste of time? What if it's a huge disappointment? What if I don't make it?" This line of questioning can go on and on ad nauseam, to the point where we can't make ANY decision at all and become stuck in hesitancy and inertia. At this point, what we really need to do is:

Set sail with a curious attitude.

Doesn't that feel nice just to say those words? Can you feel the pressure lifted? It's still a moving forward but gently, steadily and with quiet enthusiasm.

So, you see that island again off in the distance and you think, "Hmm, I wonder what it's like. It *might* be promising." And this time, the simple curiosity is all you need at this moment to leave port!

From this new, vast perspective aboard your vessel, you see another island on the starboard side. "Wow," you think, "that island looks even better!" So, from the helm, you tack and jibe towards your new destination, feeling a sense of hope and freedom even greater than the first island provided. And you are *definitely* happier than when you were in port.

Here's the point (and I know you've already figured it out): You would never have gotten to that amazing second (or third or fourth or fifth) island if you had never left the port. But by setting sail with curiosity, you headed into the open ocean with a spring in your sail and an eye for adventure. And you made sure to look around in all directions and enjoy the whole voyage.

So, like a radical fad diet or an ultra-extreme workout, even if you had burst forth from port, paddling furiously with goal-oriented tunnel vision towards that one island, you would not have seen all that was around you and perhaps would have gotten exhausted and given up.

So "set sail" with curiosity. You just may find that by simply beginning the journey to health, you'll open up a whole new world of wellness for yourself!

THE PHYSICAL HOUSE

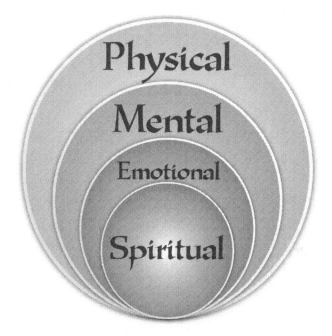

W hen I use the term *Physical House*, I mean the body itself, the part of "us" that is objectively measurable: our weight, blood pressure, heart and lungs, etc. At first glance, compared to the other three, the *Physical House* should be the easiest to diagnose and the easiest to change, but it oftentimes is a perplexing puzzle. A perfect example is weight gain and weight loss.

You have no doubt seen many celebrities in the news *trying* to take weight off (it is well publicized and glamorized) and they do so successfully, then six months later, find themselves back to their original size (or even bigger). Why is this?

One reason for rebound weight gain is because of the misapplication and misuse of goal setting that we spoke about earlier. Another explanation is because that celebrity oftentimes is using only a Physical House approach to address a multi-House problem, one that is not just physical, but also emotional, mental and spiritual. If you are trying to stop an addictive behavior such as overeating, you cannot simply *just eat less* and be successful. With the way weight loss drugs and weight loss programs advertise the situation, it seems really easy to accomplish, but anyone who has tried simply to limit their caloric intake, without any other support, knows the real truth.

"Environment is stronger than willpower."

-Paramahansa Yogananda,
Indian yogic master and author

By "environment," Yogananda is not simply referring to where you live and work, although this is important. He is also referring to the environment of your mind (the Mental House), the emotional environment of your relationships (the Emotional House) and on the deepest level, the environment of your spirit (the Spiritual House). To make weight loss permanent, it takes a powerful combination of psychological attitude change, a thorough process of revealing and healing emotional wounds and trauma, and perhaps most importantly, a positive, disciplined *inner* spiritual environment.

So, if you are on the same page with me, and agree that these are all critically necessary for a successful weight loss program, imagine what needs to happen to stay well after a bout with cancer. You might think that there is a lot more to do and that it may be much more complex, but in reality, *it is the same process.* The goal of health is the same no matter what starting point we begin at, whether it is cancer, obesity, or whatever illness we have. As I said earlier, there are many diseases, but only one "health."

The reason that I have championed an integrative approach like the "Houses of Health" is because regardless of the health issue, the basic formula fundamentally fits for all: we need to look at all four houses to achieve a real, lasting healing. The process simply needs to be tweaked and refined for each person and their specific problem. Understanding this is critically important to lasting health!

Within the *Physical House*, there are three main components that need to be examined closely: Nutrition, Sleep and Exercise. If you have a problem with any one or more of these areas, you are probably already well aware of it. But let's delve deeper into the specific factors that play into each component, as well as examine the research behind each recommendation.

NUTRITION

For those of you who are new to exploring the concept of nutrition, this simple approach may seem surprisingly easy and comforting. For those of you already well along on your healing journey, this information may seem elementary and perhaps even unsophisticated to you but bear with me. *Complex* does not necessarily mean *better.* And even the things you may already know are worth reviewing and cementing into your mind. And who knows, maybe you'll even learn something new. I know whenever I say, "I already know this," I end up learning something when I continue on with an open mind.

The Secret to Healthy Eating: Eat What You Are

You have no doubt heard this quote before: "You are what you eat." If I look back on my life and recall my eating habits of the past, I can start to feel pretty awful about all the sugar-laden junk food, deep-fried delicacies and cancer causing, chargrilled meats I've consumed in my lifetime. So, I flipped the script from "you are what you eat" which can be disheartening and disempowering to *"eat what you are"* which endows us with common sense and optimism.

What are we? Living beings. Alive. Vital. Essential. Because of this truth, the guiding principle that I teach to all my patients is to "eat things that are alive, primarily fruits, vegetables and nuts." People ask me, "what about meats?" There is ample research showing that vegetarians live an average of about 10-20% longer than non-vegetarians.[xi] I personally am not a strict vegetarian, but my diet is mostly vegetarian and dairy-free. I do believe that if meats are to be consumed, they should still be consumed with the same intention: baked, steamed or boiled as opposed to burnt or fried.

What about things that don't require refrigeration? I'm not talking about fruits, vegetables and nuts here. I am referring to what are called "shelf-stable" foods, meaning products that have been processed so that they can be safely stored at room temperature in a sealed container for countless years.

Think about this for a moment. If a food product sits on a shelf for three years and it *tastes exactly the same* as when it was put on the shelf, how good do you think it is for you? Again, common sense and easy to remember:

Eat what you are. You are alive.

Connections Between the Houses

As we discussed earlier, all of the Houses of Health are connected–the Physical, Mental, Emotional and Spiritual.

So, for example, if you are having issues trying to change your diet take a look at this particular area from the perspective of each of the Houses: (Circle any issues that feel appropriate to you.)

Physically: What are the physical issues facing you with regard to changing your diet? (These may include obesity, high blood sugar levels, poor muscular strength, low endurance, poor cardiovascular health, unexplained pain, poor flexibility, abnormal vital signs, low nutrition knowledge, lack of exercise, low or too high amount of sleep, poor quality of sleep, insomnia, sleep apnea.)

_____

_____

How engaged are you in your own physical wellness?

_____

Mentally: What are the psychological issues facing you with regard to changing your diet? (These may include poor stress management, unhealthy coping behaviors, low self-esteem, lack of willpower, lack of discipline, no sense of direction, low mental energy, anxiety, anger, confusion, persistent thoughts and/or memories, hearing voices, obsessive-compulsive tendencies, negative thoughts and affirmations, poor attitude, irritable personality.)

_____

_____

How engaged are you in your own mental wellness?

_____

_____

Emotionally: What are the emotional issues facing you with regard to changing your diet? (These may include low motivation, low self-worth, low self-esteem, social with-drawal, blunted expressive behavior, psycho-physiological changes, cultural differences and customs that are hard to go against, fighting with family or friends, mood swings, unresolved feelings, anger, apathy, confidence, curiosity, despair, envy, euphoria, fear, grief, hatred, jealousy, loneliness, lust, pity, pride, satisfaction, shock, shyness, numbness, depression.)

_____

_____

How engaged are you in your own emotional wellness?

_____

_____

Spiritually: What are the spiritual issues facing you with regard to changing your diet? (These may include anger toward a higher power, negative religious programming, despondency about the meaning of life, fear of death or afterlife, extreme ideas about reward and punishment, lack of trust, shame, lack of passion, unhappiness.)

_____

_____

How engaged are you in your own spiritual wellness?

_____

_____

As you explored each of the Houses, did you find yourself feeling down or despondent because of all the issues? Did you find yourself resisting even wanting to try? Give yourself a break! This type of resistance is normal and a part of being human when a new idea is presented to the consciousness. Be patient, compassionate and forgiving with your "flaws." Give yourself the encouragement and freedom to improve gradually and steadily. Remember: One small step at a time, my friend! Kaizen!

And also, make sure to be gentle with yourself if/when you stumble. Missteps and slide backs are all part of the process. There is no doubt that change will bring up all kinds of scary and wonderful discoveries from inside you. But if you approach it all with non-judgment, hope and your own sense of innate curiosity, you can really enjoy the ride and cement subtle but lasting changes.

My Bestselling Diet Book

I often joke that my diet book would be a nightmare for publishers, because it would only have one chapter in it. From speaking with many patients and friends making dietary changes, they are often following too many rules and plans that are extraordinarily radical. When someone declares to me, "I did a ten-day liquid diet!" I am impressed from a "WOW" standpoint, that someone could go ten days without solid food, but that's not really health. Why? It's because the habits of behavior didn't really change in a lasting way in those ten days. It was an act of will- an impressive act- but not anything that would dramatically change that person's body or health for the long term. Think back to a radical diet you committed to for physical goals. Most likely you are NOT still doing it!

The basic takeaway I am trying to get through to you is to keep it simple. Use your common sense, guided by some simple suggestions such as the ones below. What we are looking for is lasting change, a plan you can easily do *for the rest of your life.*

"The most successful people in the world make all decisions with the long term in mind."

-Paraphrased from Brian Tracy,
businessman and author

How to Know What to Eat at the Supermarket (Perimeter Shopping)

I call it Perimeter Shopping for one simple reason: You can mostly eat the foods "on the perimeter" of the supermarket to be healthy. Why? Because that's usually where the refrigeration units are. Pretty much anything that requires refrigeration means it can spoil or rot, which means it's alive. (Remember? Eat what you are, you're alive!) That means that there is a very good chance that it is okay to eat. This includes meats (not red), vegetables, fruits and the salad bar. CHEATER'S NOTE: Keep in mind, if a supermarket designed its store to have the ice cream and frozen pizza section on the "perimeter," that doesn't mean, "Dr. Roy said it was okay!"

So, let's look at what is usually NOT on the perimeter of the supermarket: boxed crackers, potato chips, sodas, candy, canned goods, and heavily processed foods. Don't fool yourself into thinking these selections are healthy. Most of them are loaded with preservatives, sugar, and ingredients you can't even pronounce.

What about frozen foods? The frozen food section often cuts straight through the middle of the store and this is intentional because these are the most tempting and "convenient" meals. More recently I have seen companies that specialize in healthy convenient options, but many are just convenient and not healthy at all. Check the packaging ingredients.

If you learned nothing else about nutrition for the rest of your life, you could survive by Perimeter Shopping and your life would still change for the better. Why? For two reasons: 1. Perimeter Shopping is a decent, easy-to-remember guideline that will mostly keep you out of trouble. 2. The more important reason is that most supermarkets put "whole foods" on the perimeter. What are whole foods? We are not talking about the supermarket *Whole Foods*. We are talking about foods that are un-processed and unrefined. These foods are the way Mother Nature created them and not coincidentally, our bodies do the best with them, digestion and absorption wise. So, if you want to keep things as simple as possible and not get overwhelmed by the overload of information out there, let Perimeter Shopping guide you gently to better health. It has worked for me and I know it will work for you to get you back on the right track.

Ten Guidelines (Not Commandments) of Eating

IMPORTANT NOTE: If your doctor has recommended a dietary restriction for a specific disease or health condition that differs from the following guidelines, FOLLOW YOUR DOCTOR'S ORDERS, not these guidelines! These are written for those readers without specific restrictions. Examples would be people with clotting disorders who cannot have a diet that is rich in dark leafy greens (as it exacerbates the condition), or people who have nut allergies cannot use almond milk (as it may cause life threatening reactions). There are many others, so please use your common sense and also follow your doctor's orders!

If you are reading this and are chomping at the bit for more specific information, I am including this section, somewhat reluctantly. Again, I really want you to keep it simple, but I also realize that some of you are already eating fresh whole foods and want things to bump it up a notch. Now remember, these are not hard and fast rules written in stone. Rather, these are suggestions that are worth your health to experiment with.

NEW HABIT FORMATION TIP: Pick only ONE of these that feels reasonable and easy for you to do for ten weeks. Resolve to do this one thing, every day. Get people on board with you as your support team!

I. Thou Shalt Try to Avoid Preservatives.

If you start reading labels, you'll find that pretty much anything that isn't refrigerated has a preservative in it. A preservative "preserves" things. This means that foods that "die" in a certain timeframe are not allowed to expire. This forces the food to remain in a pattern that isn't natural.

Physical to Emotional Connection: If you think about this in terms of "cancer as a form of resentment," as we discussed earlier, it makes sense. What is resentment? Resentment is a preserved negative mental and emotional pattern that we won't let go of. We certainly don't want our food to remain in an unnatural pattern. If the food wasn't "designed" by nature to live past its innate expiration date, putting this preservative into our bodies helps to create a passive environment where "emotional preservation" can occur.

II. Thou Shalt TRY to Avoid Refined Sugar and
    High Fructose Corn Syrup.

Cancer loves sugar. In fact, in cancer diagnosis, we use sugar to detect cancer. In PET scanning, we actually *label* a sugar molecule with a fluorescent particle (FDG Glucose) that goes right to tumors. Why? High turnover cells like cancer pick up the sugar molecule and use it preferentially over other metabolically slower tissues. Even though other highly active tissues compete with the cancer for nutrients, the cancer is usually the winner.

High fructose corn syrup is basically liquid sugar. If that wasn't bad enough, it is also made from corn, a crop known to have a lot of genetic modifications to it. Here is a convincing reason to avoid it as best you can:

In 2014, the World Health Organization recommended that the amount of sugar a person takes in daily be less than 5% of the total daily energy intake. This roughly amounts to about six teaspoons a day. Guess how many teaspoons are in just one can of soda. Nine![xii]

III. *Thou Shalt make a rainbow in thy food basket.*

Buy "colorful" fruits and veggies when you shop. Take a look at the fruit and vegetable section. You'll see greens (kale, spinach, broccoli), whites (cauliflower, onion, garlic) purples (avocado, carrots), reds (strawberries, apples), orange (carrot, turmeric), checkered (mushrooms). Not coincidentally, if you create a rainbow of color, they will contain all the vitamins and cancer fighting nutrients you need. There are cancer busters, like broccoli, spinach, kale, etc. but this specificity isn't as necessary to remember as is the basic guideline.

IV. Thou Shalt TRY to Avoid Human Interference in Food If Possible.

By human interference, I mean artificially produced pesticides, genetic modifications, and antibiotics. The easiest way to avoid all three is to buy organic. Right now, organic is still more expensive than non-organic and this may not be possible for some readers. That gap is closing, and still I do recognize that most of us are on a budget. So, if this is an issue, it is *way* better to eat non-organic produce than not eat it at all!

Some produce contains more pesticides than others. The Environmental Working Group every year comes out with a list called, "The Dirty Dozen" which details the twelve "dirtiest" fruits and veggies that should only be consumed in their organic versions, if at all possible. (Their website is easily found on Google.) A simple guideline is that any food in which you eat the skin is better eaten organic. (e.g. apples, strawberries, grapes)

All this being said, if you are on a limited budget, eating ANY kind of fruits and vegetables, organic or not, is still *WAY* better than not having them at all.

V. Thou Shalt TRY to Avoid Artificial Sweeteners.

Artificial sweeteners are called "artificial" for a reason. Here is the dictionary definition of artificial: "made or produced by human beings rather than occurring naturally, typically as a copy of something natural." In short, these compounds are made because they are cheaper and they are meant to replicate taste-wise the natural compounds they are replacing. This "commandment" is a no-brainer. Our brains and palates are often addicted to the sweetness. It has been shown that the body is fooled into thinking that this sweetness is representative of nutrition.[xiii] We also do not know the effect these artificial sweeteners have on our long-term health, because it has not been studied. I personally do not add any sweetener into anything, drinking unsweetened tea over any sweetened products. (I know, this is a sacrilegious concept in the South!) It takes some time to get used to but I prefer it now. If you do require sweeteners, in order of preference I would choose: Raw Honey (which is usually solid at room temperature) followed by Sucanat (a raw evaporated cane sugar), followed by evaporated cane sugar, followed by blackstrap molasses, followed by Stevia and xylitol.

VI. Thou Shalt TRY to Limit or Eliminate Wheat Consumption.

My one big "rule" when I'm thinking about healthy food is, "Could I eat it raw?" Meaning, "Can it be eaten unprocessed?" Fruits? Yes. Veggies? Yes. Meat? Yes. (Sushi, steak tartar, etc.) Wheat? No. It needs to be pounded, processed and baked. Why is this an issue? Well, your body isn't made to process it naturally. The wheat has to be modified to be processed by the gut.

Many people who have "stomach issues," may find, at closer look, that they actually have either a gluten sensitivity issue or simply just a wheat digestion issue. (People with a disease called Celiac Disease have a true intolerance and will get very sick if they ingest any wheat gluten.) If this could be a possibility, you don't need a blood test per se, but rather, just try to stop eating it for two weeks and see how you feel. Look around and you'll start seeing all the "gluten-free" products popping up, some healthy, some not. So, there are options out there but look closely and choose wisely.

Some who are skeptical about the linkage between gut health and wheat point out that Celiac Disease, which is a true intolerance to wheat gluten, only exists in a small percentage of people. I think their misunderstanding is in the fact that there is a difference between intolerance, allergy and sensitivity. Intolerance is a true bodily inability to digest- producing nausea and vomiting almost immediately, as is the case with Celiac Disease. Allergy is having the ability to process but once processed causes a bodily reaction, like a rash, or shortness of breath. Sensitivity is having the ability to process but also having a more insidious and possibly time delayed symptom complex, such as fatigue or stomach pain. In my case, for example, I have a dairy allergy; I get rashes and even nosebleeds due to eating it. I also have a corn sensitivity. If corn is processed, like in tortilla chips, it gives me a lot of upset stomach symptoms. However, if it is in its natural form (corn on the cob) I can eat it just fine.

VII. Thou Shalt build in a reward meal.

You can be really disciplined with your eating habits, but let's be compassionate with it. Why? Because we are looking to set goals that we can maintain for life, not just a few weeks. When people comment to me, "Wow, you are strict with that food stuff!" I correct them, saying I follow "most of it, most of the time, but not all of it, all the time." When I decide to choose something unhealthy, it's usually in the fried potato family: potato chips, French fries, tater tots... I could go on, but I won't! I'll eat these once in a while even though I know that they are high in saturated fats (not good for my heart) and also that fried food contains acrylamide, a byproduct of high heat cooking which has been shown to be carcinogenic (also present in baked foods, FYI). My point in telling you this is that letting go of the leash for a bit gives me psychological freedom. I can be 100% strict for a few weeks, but I can be 90% strict for years. And *that's* the key.

VIII. Thou Shalt drastically reduce or cut out dairy consumption.
(Dairy: Milk, Cheese, and Butter)

Why cut it out? Well, first consider this fact: Aside from the Red-billed Oxpecker, a bird lives in the Amazon, *humans are the only animals on the planet that drink the milk of another animal.* We have the enzyme for digesting cow's milk as children but more than 75% of adults lose the expression of that enzyme[xiv]. The one population which is able to process dairy as adults are Northwest Europeans, which of course is a large part of the US population genetically. Being that the United States is a cultural melting pot, many people from dairy intolerant parts of the world (Asia, Latin America, Africa) immigrate here and begin to eat more like the land they arrived in, and part of that is eating more dairy.

Dairy marketing has trained our minds to think that dairy is actually good for us. When I was growing up, it was "good for your bones." "Got calcium?" The milk advertisement would ask--and we have all seen the ads of famous people with a "milk moustache." Unfortunately, if you look at the science, milk (and calcium from milk) actually does not protect bone health, and in fact some studies have linked it to increased fractures[xv]. This fact alone should give those people who are prone to osteoporosis pause. Add to this the research linking dairy consumption to testicular, prostate,[xvi] and possibly to ovarian cancer,[xvii] and you get to see why dairy may not be as good for you as once thought. (Interestingly, milk advertising has switched to "Got Protein?" as their slogan now. It does have quite a bit of protein, which is why whey, which is made from milk, is a major additive for protein supplement products.)

Personally, I have completely eliminated dairy from my diet. This was no small feat, as I was so in love with cheese that I used to bring *my own Parmigiano-Reggiano* to Italian restaurants because their table grated Parmesan cheese was not up to my standards! What was happening to my body? I had started to get a lot of stomach pain, loose bowel movements, and fatigue. I knew that I might have been lactose intolerant already (95% of people of Asian descent are) so I started to take lactase pills with each dairy-filled meal to help digest the dairy. This relieved most of my symptoms, so I thought, "well, thank God I can have my freshly grated cheese!" Unfortunately, over the next few years, I began to get unexplainable rashes on my lower back, armpit and lip. I visited a few doctors who told me they thought I might have a fungal infection, and I was recommended to take an antifungal medication for six months. This did not sound right to me. Eventually I went to see Dr. Eve Campanelli, who is an herbalist and naturopathic practitioner. I told her about my rashes, and also mentioned that I had a lot of "seasonal allergies" that got pretty severe, sneezing, eye itching, and even with nosebleeds sometimes. I also mentioned I got sick quite frequently, maybe 6-8 times a year.

She listened and then asked me politely, "Do you eat a lot of dairy?"

My answer was an anxious question. "You don't think all this is from dairy, do you?" She nodded but said not much more on the subject. After a fruitful visit, I got herbs to support my immune system, which I was happy about because of the illnesses I had been getting. Also, when I left the office, I promptly forgot about her telling me to stop dairy!

When I returned a few months later, the rashes had not let up. She asked me again, "Did you stop dairy?" I was shocked and paused. I shook my head 'no' sheepishly but inwardly I knew I had to stop. Since that day in 2009, I have totally cut out all dairy, and I am glad to say that all my rashes have gone away, and that my "seasonal allergies" have almost completely gone away, and my number of sicknesses per year have gone down to 1-2 times per year.

IX. Thou Shalt Cut Down or Eliminate Red Meat Consumption.

Sorry folks. I hate to do it. I really do. Just so you know, I'm from Buffalo, the land of Beef-on-Weck, Prime Rib specials, AND I lived in Philadelphia for five years, home of the Philly Cheesesteak, AND I live now in Los Angeles, a major hub for Korean and Japanese foods that feature marinated beef kalbi and slow-cooked pork, so I know exactly the implications of what I'm writing here. There are multiple studies[xviii] correlating the association of red meat with an increase in cancer, in some studies as high as 20% for killers such as lung and esophageal cancer.[xix] There are multiple studies that show a vegetarian diet improves overall survival. [xx]

Of course, there are those meat-eating advocates who state that the effect of "bad red meat" i.e. processed with hormones, fed on corn-based diets instead of grass, will reduce negative effects of eating red meat. This may have some truth in it, however until the sourcing of beef and pork is "clean" for everyone and shows that the red meat itself wasn't the culprit, I will recommend for red meat's reduction or removal from diets.

X. Thou Shalt Make 50% of My Diet Green.

The first thing I ask when I talk to people about improving their diets is the following question: "How much of your diet is green?" By "green" I mean salads, vegetables or fruits (of any color). It may be imprecise, because fruits and vegetables are all the colors of the rainbow, but it gets the point across, and it serves as a simple reminder to eat more vegetables and fruits. In fact, the US Government's recommendation (through USDA's MyPlate.gov website) recommends half of each meal's plate should be either fruits or vegetables![xxi] This is surprising to me, as I would normally assume the government would be behind the times, but it just goes to show us how important "eating green" is. From my own informal surveys, less than 25% of people actually do meet this recommendation

Also, as I stated earlier in Commandment IX, there are studies that have shown that completely "non-meat" diets, including vegetarian or vegan, are the ones with the strongest data of increasing overall lifespan.

XI. (BONUS COMMANDMENT)
Thou Shalt Not Overly Emphasize Nutrition!

Every talk I give, I leave room for questions at the end. It has been a consistent pattern that the vast majority of questions asked are about nutrition. This isn't a bad thing and it's not that nutrition isn't important. What I think the pattern demonstrates is the mind's need to find something it can identify and change in a concrete way. Nutrition fits that mold. "Sugar is bad? OK. Check! I can stop that and feel better!" Don't get me wrong: I think trying to improve one's eating habits is very important, but I have too often seen that the other Houses (Emotional, Mental, Spiritual) are avoided. The intention to be healthier by diet alone is really masking a strong desire to avoid feeling any pain through the uncovering of deeper, harder to perceive, unhealthy habits. So, if this fits you, continue reading on before starting any diet change. There might be a more important thing to look at and change!

What Can I Eat??!

Just a reminder, although we jokingly called these commandments, they are simply guidelines to consider. Additionally, if you decide to remove things, especially sugar or dairy, remember that you are cutting out a lot of calories. In my case, when I first tried to remove dairy, I did not think about *what to add in*. This is very important. We do need a certain number of calories, including fats and proteins. This is not a diet book, so I am not going to get into calorie counts or nutritional planning. These resources can be found online if you are looking to see what calories you are taking in. A nutritionist who is experienced with cancer or whichever disease you are working through can really be helpful. I would suggest an integrative nutritionist, someone who sees a 'holistic' view of food as a part of a larger approach like the Houses of Health. I did meet with a nutritionist a few times to get my bearings and it was really helpful.

Specific Foods That Are Shown to Be "Anti-Cancer"

What I would call a balanced idea of eating is "plant-centered," not "plant only." A plant-centered diet is consistent with all the above ten recommendations. As for specific foods to eat, I hesitate somewhat to offer this advice, simply because it is human nature to buy these foods and say, "Well, I'm covered!" That being said, I think there is a value to knowing that you are *including* the right foods. This list could be much longer; these are just the ones I have found evidence for by the time of publication and also were the most important in my opinion.

One easy way to start is to eat one food from each column each day. That way, you'll know that you have gotten some "immune boosters" and "cancer fighters" into your system the way you were supposed to always be getting them: by eating them.

SALAD STUFF	SMELLY STUFF	FINGER FOODS
Broccoli,	**Beans**	**Cranberries**
Spinach	**Leeks**	**Acai Berries**
Kale	**Onions**	**Blueberries**
Watercress	**Garlic**	**Seeds**
Cabbage		**Strawberries**
Romaine Lettuce		**Walnuts**
Collard Greens		
Brussel Sprout		

FUNGI & FERMENTED		DRINKABLES
Mushrooms:		**Green Tea**
White button, Shitake		**Kombucha Kefir**
Portobello, Crimini		**Ginger Tea**
Fermented:		
Tempeh, Miso,		
Soy Sauce		
(preferably Tamari,		
non-wheat soy sauce)		

Lose That Tire!

Now that we have gone over what to eat, let's actually look at *eating* itself. All over the industrialized world, we are experiencing an explosion in obesity. A full 70% of the United States' population over 20 years old is either overweight or obese.[xxii] There are multiple studies showing that caloric restriction actually improves survival from cancer. In fact, it improves health for all categories of disease. I know caloric restriction isn't as sexy or exciting as the recent diet your friend is doing on Facebook or what Dr. Oz recommends, but it certainly is more budget-friendly and requires only one quality to get it started: self-discipline. (Sometimes spending money is easier, I know.)

The evidence pointing to being overweight as a risk factor for cancer is well-documented in the literature. Obese people have higher cancer rates and recurrence rates, especially kidney, colon, breast, esophageal and endometrial cancers.[xxiii] Additionally, every 30 pounds of weight increases cancer mortality by 10%. [xxiv]

Why would being overweight be a risk factor? Within the body, it has been shown that important signaling molecules, IGF-1 and IGF-1R, are lowered with caloric restriction.[xxv] Both of these have been shown in animal models to increase tumor growth and also decrease the effectiveness of cancer therapies. In studies of radiation therapy, IGF-1 levels have been shown to rise significantly right after treatment, likely induced by the cancer to protect itself!

As a crossover to the Spiritual House, the ancient spiritual masters who advocated fasting for spiritual reasons probably also knew this was good for the body itself. Buddhism, Hinduism, Islam, Judaism, and Christianity have aspects of fasting that are still followed today. Even in America where fasting is not practiced as much, we see some glimpses of this in the giving up of certain foods for Yom Kippur, Lent and Ramadan, for example. Even God rested for a day, thus it makes sense for the human digestive system to rest as well. I personally have done periods where I fast one day a week, usually on the weekend, only having fresh squeezed orange juice with blended almonds and copious amounts of water. This allows my gut to rest and I do notice an increased calmness and lower rate of stomach issues because of it.

(Caveat: People who are post-cancer treatment who have experienced profound weight loss (called cachexia) should NOT attempt caloric restriction, as they may be malnourished. Even in these populations, it has been shown that the weight loss is from an aggressive tumor, rather than not eating enough. Even so, these people should contact a nutritionist if caloric restriction is an appealing strategy.)

The Role of the Microbiome in Immunity

The microbiome is the community of microorganisms that live in our bodies, which include bacteria, viruses, yeasts, and more. In Los Angeles where the health industry is front and center, people often ask me about the role of probiotics in one's health. A probiotic can be defined as a "live microorganism which, when consumed regularly, provides a beneficial health effect on the body."[xxvi] Basically, a probiotic is a "good bacteria" added to your gut, whereas the microbiome is the whole population, added or existing. In Los Angeles, if you go to the supermarket or turn on the TV, you will see the word "probiotics" all over the place: on yogurt labels, on pill bottles, and if you are really in the know, you have heard about it in live fermented foods, like raw sauerkraut or Korean kimchi. The question becomes, is it harmful to knowingly add bacteria to your body? And if it is not harmful, does it really help?

Bacteria in the collective consciousness are usually branded as bad, which is the result of good marketing by the antibacterial soap companies. It makes sense on one level- you don't want unwanted pathogens in your body. The intestinal tract is a little different though, because it's actually more like the *outside* of your body rather than the inside, being that it's connected to the outside world like your skin on the front end (your mouth) and the back end (your anus). Also, unbeknownst to most of us, we have more bacteria in our intestines (called "gut flora") than human cells in our bodies, by a ratio of 1.3:1. [xxvii] So it's not that we are introducing something "new" into our bodies: They've always been there, populating our bodies since birth until now. You may ask, how about when a baby is in the womb? As a fetus in the womb, it is a sterile environment, meaning having no bacteria present. When a baby is born, the gut begins to populate with bacteria.

The problem is, due to poor nutritional habits combined with life stressors, the gut can become unhealthy and the ratio of good to bad bacteria can become unbalanced.

A very well-known example would be the bacteria known as *H.Pylori*, which has been shown to be causative in gastric disease, such as peptic ulcers. Doctors frequently prescribe antibiotics to destroy it. Unfortunately, this also kills the good bacteria as well, and a healthy homeostasis (internal balance) may be hard to reestablish. I have a friend who had to go through the *H.Pylori* antibiotic regimen and felt, "Whew! I am glad *that's* gone." He called me as he started having loose stools after the antibiotic course. We started him on a probiotic that helped to regulate his bowel movements.[xxviii] He also started to implement new habits as well, because going back to the same eating habits and life stressors would only set himself up for a reemergence of *H.Pylori* and subsequently the ulcer issue. You might ask, why don't we just eliminate *H.Pylori* in everyone? The reason is in balanced individuals *H.Pylori's* presence is protective against Barrett's esophagus, which is a precursor to esophageal cancer.[xxix] So again, it's the balance of the microbiome that is important.

The World Health Organization has started the process of looking at studies that address what things are helped by probiotics. [xxx] It's not a new idea, just one that has started to gain traction. The first report of a probiotic effect was in 1907, by a scientist named Tissier. Moreover, in Eastern Europe, *kefir,* which contains a culture of Lactobacillus, has been consumed daily as a healthy (and tasty) beverage prior to even that time, being recommended as early as the late 1800's.

The Microbiome and Cancer

The million-dollar question is whether these probiotics can help protect the body from diseases like cancer. I think the data, although emerging, provides some encouraging evidence that probiotics indirectly affect cancer by improving the immune system, through their effect on allergies in infants,[xxxi] for example, and directly in exciting research in bladder cancer and colon cancer.[xxxii] In some very intriguing research, a recently published paper showed in mice that these "good bacteria" naturally present in the gut were crucial to the delivery of chemotherapy during treatment.[xxxiii] In this mouse study published in the highly regarded journal *Science,* it was seen that gut bacteria travelled through the gut wall into the lymph nodes to help stimulate the immune system, which allowed the chemotherapy to be more effective. Mice who were treated with antibiotics prior to chemotherapy (thereby eradicating its normal gut flora) showed tumor resistance to the chemotherapy.

It is no surprise to find that the microbiome makeup extends even more than just to a local effect in the gut. Studies are emerging, again in mice models, which demonstrate that the health of your gut bacteria can affect your metabolism.[xxxiv] Researchers found that if they transplanted the gut bacteria from an obese mouse to a thin mouse, gave them the same diet, the thin mouse became obese. When they transplanted the thin mouse flora to the obese mouse, the obese mouse became thinner.

Although these findings are tantalizing and need to be replicated in humans, a more important (but less marketed) factor in microbiome health is what are called *prebiotics.* Prebiotics are the food that healthy gut bacteria need to eat to grow. This includes but isn't limited to foods such as jicama, unripe bananas, onions, garlic, asparagus, barley and oatmeal. If you modify your diet to include more raw plants overall you will naturally be giving your microbiome the nutrition it needs. In surprising new research coming out, there is some suggestion that if your food choices are unhealthy, it may be the "bad bacteria" driving your food choices by sending signals to your brain to eat the things *they* like! [xxxv] Talk about a conspiracy!

Physical to Mental House Crossover

One of the main goals of this book is to highlight the ways in which each House affects the other Houses. Along this line of thinking, researchers working with mice found that the bacterial inhabitants of the gut can affect the levels of calmness or anxiety seen in the mice.[xxxvi] They found that by adding certain helpful bacteria to the gut of mice, anxious mice were transformed into more fearless mice, due to a change in neurotransmitter function. This is fascinating, as I think most of us would *not* give bacteria any credit to change the state of mind of any being, whether mouse or man! Again, these are mice studies, but just the fact that this research *exists* makes me feel that the microbiome carries an untapped potential.

You may ask what I do. Personally, I drink a probiotic drink 2-3 times a week. I even got into it so much that for a few years I "home brewed" the above-mentioned kefir, to get my daily dose of probiotics. I did this at home because it's cheaper than buying a store-bought brand (which can be $4-$6 per serving), and also because I like to take ownership of my own health. Plus, it's fun to make different flavors, experiment with them, and then see the weird faces that friends make when I tell them what it is. (They eventually try it, and some of them even like it!)

SLEEP

"Getting a good night's sleep is fairly simple, if you allow yourself to do it. The big problem for cancer patients is they take too much on themselves and don't give enough time to help their bodies cope with the illness. They're worried about burdening their families and fulfilling their usual obligations."

— Dr. David Spiegel, Ph.D. researcher

Despite the fact that sleep takes up a quarter to a third of our lives, the purpose of sleep is not well understood by scientists. However, one thing that is *easily* understood by everyone, researcher or not: *we need it to function well.* We intuitively know that we feel more energetic, happier, more peaceful, and feel like we can handle all things that come to us when we have a good night's sleep. However, there is a disconnect somewhere between what we know and what we do, isn't there? If sleep does all these wonderful things, then why do most of us *not* get enough of it? (The Centers for Disease Control estimated in 2016 that a third of Americans do not get the recommended 7 hours of sleep per night.)

Emotional to Mental House Crossover: Childhood

From my point of view, getting enough sleep has a strong Emotional House component to it. Oftentimes, when we were kids, we were forced to go to bed when we didn't want to, often kicking and screaming. Does this sound familiar? If so, there may be an old childhood pattern of being stubborn and fighting what is good for us with what we feel like doing. It also goes back to *love*. Was bedtime made special by your parents? Did they make it an event? Reading a story together? Or did they watch TV, stay downstairs and say to you, "Go to bed now!" This would trigger a feeling of loss, separation anxiety, or abandonment that would and could and probably did traumatize that time before bed, creating that familiar, "I don't want to go to bed yet!" feeling inside. Now, imagine if bedtime were made a loving event, maybe a time where parent and child got to bond. It might have you feeling excited to go to bed! This creates a habit pattern in the brain of something good.

Another thing to consider: Do we like what we are going to wake up to in the morning? Remember that feeling on Sunday as a kid, before school started again on Monday? Not a great feeling, right? Now flash forward to today: If one *hates* his or her job, why would we want to go to bed to go to it the next day? I wouldn't. A figurative (and literal) wake-up call is necessary.

Just this realization can help us, as we can take better care of ourselves around bedtime. We need to reestablish a positive feeling before we go to bed. Take the time to surround yourself with things you like to do, that make you feel loved. Then you might want to go to bed *earlier* to experience this feeling!

On the other end, insomnia can cause extreme anxiety about going to bed. It is a frustrating thing to experience, and if you have ever had it, you know it can cause a sense of hopelessness even if you only have it for a short period of time. Thus, if you can't fall asleep, it makes sense that you would avoid trying. How to combat it? Read on!

The Evidence for the Importance of Sleep

As with any other issue, researchers see improvement when we educate the adult brain on specifically *why* sleep is good for you. This increases the wisdom component of the equation. So, it becomes a balanced choice- "Do I stay up and sleep five hours because I want to watch TV (short-term fix)? Or do I go to bed earlier knowing that I will be happier tomorrow and healthier overall (long-term happiness)?"

Research shows that sleep:

1. Extends your life: Multiple studies demonstrate that people who sleep less than 5 hours have a 15% shorter life expectancy than those who sleep more than 6 hours.[xxxvii]

2. Clears out neural toxins, allowing the brain to "detox." The tiredness you feel is oftentimes a sign the brain needs to shut down to recoup.[xxxviii]

3. Increases your immunity. People who sleep more have more resistance to infections.^{xxxix}

4. Decreases your weight. People who sleep less than six hours have a higher Body Mass Index (a weight to height ratio) than those who sleep more. ^{xl}

5. Makes you happier and less prone to mood disorders like depression.

How to Get a Good Night's Sleep

I had a lot of periods of insomnia growing up, so I have taken this issue really seriously and did my best to set myself up for success with sleep. It really is a Four House process:

Physical House: I make sure I exercise regularly to burn off excess energy, every day if possible. I avoid caffeine late in the day, and better yet, avoid it completely. I find that even if I drink one caffeinated beverage after noontime, it either makes going to sleep tougher or it makes me wake up in the middle of the night for no apparent reason. I avoid high fructose corn syrup and sugary foods after dinner.

Mental House: I really made "doing what I love" a priority. This was a big thing for me. As I mentioned in the Introduction, I didn't feel like I was fulfilled in my life. If that is the case for you, and you're not taking any steps towards an inner feeling of fulfillment, it makes sense that the unconscious part of ourselves feels like it has a right to cause issues, whether by insomnia or making us not sleep enough.

Emotional House: If there are unresolved issues emotionally that remain buried, it makes sense that those issues can indirectly cause insomnia. I did a lot of therapy to unearth these issues and not surprisingly my sleep steadily improved.

Spiritual House: Personally, I have four things I do on a nightly basis. I do a meditation before I go to bed, something that is proven to lower anxiety and increase a sense of well-being. (This will be fully explored in the Spiritual House, don't worry!) Also, I have a journal there, which allows me to unpack issues from the day that I may have avoided and also process events of the day in a more complete way. The third thing is that I list five things that I am grateful for from my day, taking time to feel those feelings again if possible. The last thing I do is read a spiritual book.

Why do I do a gratitude list?

**The body does not know the difference
between feeling from a memory and
feeling the actual experience.**

If you can accept this, you can use this to your advantage. Take yourself back through great things of the day. You get a two for one! (See: Thriving vs. Languishing under the Mental House.) Finally, by reading part of a spiritual book, even if just for a minute, sets my mind in a positive frame before I actually turn the lights out. This may sound like a lot, but it can be just 15 to 20 minutes total, depending on your life situation. See what things you can build into your bedtime routine and watch your sleep improve!

EXERCISE

No surprises here! Exercise is an important part of your health. Many people ask me, "how much exercise do I have to do?" What I've found is that the people who are asking me this question usually don't exercise, or exercise very infrequently and are trying to get away with as little as possible. (If that's you, you might have an "out"! Read on!)

If you haven't built a habit throughout your life of being active, the transition time after recovery from cancer treatment, or any illness for that matter, is a GREAT opportunity. Crossing over into the Mental House, people mentally tend to associate the word "exercise" with "work." In the historical past, people used to work on their feet, so exercise wasn't so crucial. In a very real sense, exercise *was* work- they'd get their heart moving and their body moving just by going to work, either in fields or in factories, or moving around a factory, a time when a majority of the country was built on manufacturing. If you still have a job like this, where you do have a high activity level, then you're in luck! For you, work is exercise and this is protective for your immune system. You can even boost it and make it even better for yourself: I have a pediatric doctor friend who had a digital "pedometer" that recorded how much she walked and found that she walked over 7 *miles each day* while she worked. These devices are very cheap now and can be a great way to motivate yourself. My doctor friend made it even more like exercise in that she only took the stairs, which acted like a "Stairmaster" for her!

If you're not one of those who burns calories while working, it may be good to know that you are in the majority, as the United States has shifted mostly to a sedentary work culture, where most of us stand in one place or sit in front of computers for the whole day. For those of us who fit this description, we need to build a routine, to build a habit of exercise.

I grew up playing sports: basketball, tennis, swimming and golf. I also loved to weightlift because it made me feel great, gave me more strength and also made me look good. (Hey, give me a break- I was a teenager mentally, well into my twenties!) My resting heart rate was between 50-60 beats per minute. When I sprained my left knee playing basketball, I had to take four months off, and in that time my idea was, *"I'll work back my strength when my knee feels better."* That was a poor choice on my part, because when I did come back, I sprained ligaments in my *right* knee because it had been compensating for the *left* injured knee. I took *another* four months off, and when I came back to being totally "healthy," I was in terrible shape. Work began to pick up, I started choosing relationship time over workout time, and before I knew it, I had developed new habits in which I was used to a lower level of physical wellness. In fact, even four years later, I *still* had not gotten back to the pre-injury level of fitness. This was all because of a mental affirmation/attitude that crept into my mind: "I'll work myself back into shape when my knee feels better."

I tell this story so you know I have an appreciation for the difficulties of recovery. I know how much of a pain (literally and figuratively) getting back to an optimal state of wellness is, especially when one doesn't get to do what one has always done for exercise, which for me was playing full-court basketball. This four-year cycle is not unlike what one has coming off of intensive therapy for cancer (or any disease) in the sense that what you were before seems almost unattainable. Anyone who has gone through this knows exactly what I am talking about. The point is, even when one has been declared "disease-free," that's only the *start* of the process.

So, how does one combat this? How does one create a habit of exercise when nothing existed before or what was before is no more?

Habits are a Mental House thing. It may seem really subtle, but even word choice is a habit that really feels important to clarify. This is similar to sleep: I don't want to orient my mind in such a way that I use a word that has a bad feeling for me. Thus, I don't like the word "exercise." You will never hear me say, "I need to exercise," or "I'm going to exercise." These words don't inspire me to get off the couch. For me, instead of "I'm going to exercise," I like the words, "I'm going to hit the gym" or "I'm going to work out." It feels more exciting to me, and when trying to inspire yourself, *that really matters.* What I recommend in this instance can be summed up here: *Make it fun and inspiring.* If it's not fun and inspiring when I think of it, I would not do it otherwise on a regular basis; I'd choose something more fun.

Ways to make exercise more fun:

1. Work out with a partner. Someone with the same health situation as you is ideal, but also someone who has the same schedule as you may be even better. It creates accountability and makes it something to look forward to.

2. Try interactive video games, like the Nintendo Wii-fit. I know lots of people who have bought these for their kids and end up playing them themselves. It's a great way to have fun and get a workout in. For those of you with kids, you can actually play with them, plus you don't have to travel to the gym and spend that travel time.

3. Join a *convenient* gym. As we said before, "environment is stronger than willpower." The environment really helps. Sometimes when I get really tired, I still make it there and even lie on a bench for five minutes to recharge. I know if I had gone home first to rest, I never would have made it back out. Also, if you go there enough and get to know people, it can become somewhat of a social activity (as long as a workout is still done!)

4. Hire a trainer. I hired a trainer for two times a week to help me get back on track. Even if you don't have the resources to hire one full-time, you can hire them to work out with you part-time. Even once a week with someone dedicated to the craft of making your body better is an incredible help for discipline, perspective and advice. Plus, psychologically, by paying for it, you know you have to go, and over time that builds that habit!

Exercise and the Immune System

Regular exercise is *key* to your immune system's health and thus is protective against the first appearance or recurrence of cancer. Keeping with the idea that proven research is helpful to convince the brain that exercise is useful, I took a hard look at the data itself.

Thankfully I'm not the only person who values data. Much of the work was done for me: The *American Institute for Cancer Research* (World Cancer Research Fund) published an "Expert Report" in 2007[xli] in which the data for activity and cancer risk for breast, lung, pancreas, and endometrial cancers was assessed for an overall pattern. For colon cancer, the number one diagnosed invasive cancer in the United States, the evidence was *strongly* in favor of a protective effect. For postmenopausal breast cancer, and endometrial cancer, the evidence showed that exercise was probably protective. For lung, pancreas and premenopausal breast cancer, the evidence was limited, but suggestive. *Bottom line: For all of the cancers they looked at, exercise has at least some protective effect.* (Of course, as we all know, Americans can take things too far; They did not find a protective effect for extreme amounts of exercise.)

The Bonuses of Exercise

There are, as you might imagine, a lot of other benefits to exercise that aren't directly related to "cancer prevention." I mention them here to you so they can be "food for your mind" to help you motivate! Exercise has been shown to decrease your cardiac risk (of dying or having heart problems). It decreases diabetes risk (independent of decreasing obesity). It's been proven to increase bone density, which improves your bone health (and thus less risk of fractures later on). It also has been shown to improve couples' sex lives. It's also been shown to increase energy levels during the day and promote deeper, more restful sleep at night. It's also been shown to decrease in-flammation, which is also indirectly linked to cancer. It's been shown to increase *brain-derived neurotrophic factor,* which has been shown to be active in learning and memory. In another study, people over 50 who exercised regularly demonstrated better memory scores *even one year after the study ended.* [xlii]

MENTAL HOUSE CROSSOVER EXERCISE: *Right now,* take out a piece of paper and pen, and write down what positive and negative thoughts have come up around exercise. Seriously. Do it now. I'm even giving you the space to do it:

POSITIVE THOUGHTS: NEGATIVE THOUGHTS:

Now count the number of positive thoughts. Count the number of negative thoughts. See what the ratio is, positive to negative thoughts. Is it more positive than negative? Or more negative than positive? We'll talk about this more in the Mental House, but this positive to negative thought ratio is *extremely* important. If you found that there were more negatives than positives, go back up, add more on this sheet so that you create at least a 4:1 positive to negative thought ratio around exercise. (Go to the Mental House section for an in-depth discussion about the positive to negative thought ratio.)

This is a very simple exercise, but it can be done anytime to get yourself out of a rut. As we will discuss later in the Mental House section, a negative thought has twice the power of a positive thought on your actions. Thus, we have to discipline our minds and reaffirm the positive.

Obesity and Cancer

The study's authors made a significant note: The protective effect of exercise was "independent of body fatness," meaning there was an *additional* benefit for weight loss and its protective effect for cancer. The National Cancer Institute has shown that obesity is directly linked to cancer, especially for rectal, esophagus, kidney, thyroid and the ones listed above- breast, lung, and colon. [xliii] For other cancer types, including prostate (#1 diagnosed cancer in men) and ovarian cancer, being overweight is linked but not as strongly. Again, as in data on exercise, weight loss was at least linked or directly related for all cancers they looked at.

Obesity has become an epidemic in the United States right now, with over 2/3 of our citizens considered overweight or obese, with the number rising every day. To get a good sense of where one stands on this note, we simply need to look at the Body Mass Index, or BMI. Type "BMI calculator" into Google, and it will direct you to a website that has a free calculator on it. You only need your height and weight. A BMI of over 25 is considered overweight (corresponds to a body fat of 15-20%) and a BMI of over 30 is considered obese (corresponding to a body fat of 25-30%).

Take a moment to record your thoughts:

If you fit either of these, overweight or obese, did you know this information?

_____

_____

More importantly, if you are in either of these categories, how does that information make you feel?

_____

_____

Does it motivate you, or does it make you even more "stuck" and helpless?

_____

_____

The best way I have found to mentally frame any new discoveries that could be negative is to say to myself, *"It's OK, it's just information."*

This isn't a book on weight loss, but if you adjust your eating habits as suggested above, and start a minimum of exercise, and sleep enough, those habits will result in weight loss along with more energy, a better immune system and a decreased risk of cancer *without* you having to focus on it!

Sunshine on Your Shoulders

A lot of this book is designed to show you that the habits that make us healthy are very easy to do and taking in sunshine is one of them. Getting outside is fun as well. We spend so much of our time indoors, locked to our computers or the television, that we forget that what *gives us life* is the SUN. The sun provides all our energy, from the food we eat, to the electricity that powers our computers, to the gas for our cars, it all comes either directly or indirectly from the sun. We as humans also *directly* benefit from being in the sun. The body converts a cholesterol derivative into fat-soluble Vitamin D3 upon exposure to strong enough sunlight. We aren't exactly plants but not bad for organisms without chlorophyll!

For a generation trained to stay out of the sun due to cancer risk, this may be a shock: The sun is good for you, depending on *if* you live in an area that has a strong enough sun dose and *if* you dose correctly. To me this is fairly ironic: we have been worried about getting too much sun. Now we've gone the other way and are not getting enough. It's also a little bit more scientific than one might think because at least half of our country doesn't receive sunlight strong enough from November through February for Vitamin D conversion! People living at a latitude of 42 degrees north, roughly the northern California border and Boston, *do not* have sunlight that is able to convert vitamin D to its active form from November to February. This can be balanced by regular exposure to the sun during the months from April to October. Latitudes below 34 degrees north (lower than Los Angeles and Columbia, South Carolina) receive a sun dose that is adequate for vitamin D3 conversion year-round.

From a cancer perspective, yes, repeated and overly intense sun exposure is NOT a good thing. That's an obvious fact for all those people I see coming in for treatment for their skin cancers. The sun is usually strongest from approximately 10am to 2pm, and it has been advised to stay out of the sun in those times. If you need to go out during those times, using a sunblock of at least 35 SPF is recommended. Even if you live at a latitude where the sunlight is not able to do the conversion to vitamin D3, it *still* can cause cancer if there is overexposure.

Vitamin D3 is used in the body in calcium and phosphorus metabolism (good for bones). There is emerging evidence for its role in cancer and the immune system. The data has been relatively inconsistent (so far) for its effect in cancer prevention, but there is *no* study saying it's a bad thing. It's more of whether supplementing vitamin D will add anything to protect the body. A large Vitamin D/Calcium Polyp Study reported its results recently and surprisingly with Calcium and Vitamin D supplementation together, they found an *increased* risk of polyps that lead to cancer.[xliv] (Giving Vitamin D alone wasn't studied.)

NOTE: I hesitated to put this information in the book because there is no established data showing that vitamin D supplementation is effective (yet), neither is there much consensus on how much sun per day is best if one chooses to get sun exposure. I wanted to give you the information so that those of you who would consider using it to your benefit would use your best judgment and the advice of any trusted medical practitioner. For a guideline for those who are interested, the expert I found most reasonable was Dr. Michael Holick, who wrote a book called *The Vitamin D Solution.*[xlv] He recommends an amount that is based on skin type and also where you live. Obviously, if you have a history of sun damage/skin cancer or any reason that the sun may be harmful, repeated sun exposure is CLEARLY not for you!

Another way in which the sun benefits us is via the effect it has on our circadian rhythm of sleep and wake cycles. The sun is critical because it is involved in signaling the rise of cortisol and the drop in melatonin. There is no direct evidence showing that disruption of circadian clocks increase cancer, but there are studies of people who work at night, showing that they have an increased risk of cancer.[xlvi]

Our Precious Feet

We are walking around on rubber, all day, insulated from the earth. Our shoes are made to help us feel more comfortable, with ads saying, "Take care of your feet" by padding them with inserts and orthotics. This may *feel* better (and necessary for a minority of people with foot injuries) but for most of us, the reason we are having leg and foot problems in the first place is probably *because* of shoes. (Any high-heel wearers who have gone through days with their toes mashed into triangles already know this!) Our feet and ankles have muscles, ligaments and fascia that are meant to fully support our bodies. When they are in proper health they can do exactly that. When the feet are overly supported, the muscles become weak and cannot support the body. They become painful and yes, you guessed it, then you will certainly need those inserts and orthotics because the feet have failed their purpose. It's a downward spiral that we need to get out of.

Take myself for an example: I grew up being really physically active. As I got older, there was progressively less running, less activity. In the last few years I noticed my left arch started to become flat and my ankle started to hurt. First, I went to the chiropractor, who offered me orthotics to support my feet. This really helped my symptoms when I was walking. Then I noticed that without the orthotics my feet were hurting when I was playing sports (not playing 3 times a week like I used to, but once a week) so I added orthotics in those shoes. Pretty soon, I bought orthotic inserts for all my shoes. Then guess what happened? I started playing beach volleyball. You don't wear shoes in beach volleyball. So, my ankles and feet, totally deconditioned by this point, were exposed for what they really were: weak. I could barely walk the day after I played my first game! I had coincidentally hired a trainer to help me with my shoulder strength but he immediately honed in on my feet and ankles. Then I started to do exercises in bare feet that strengthened all these muscles. I'm a lot more pain free these days but I'll admit it does take *daily* awareness to remember to do these exercises. This isn't a guide to physical rehabilitation, but you can easily use Google and YouTube for free guides on foot health exercises. (Just Google "Foot health exercises" and click the "Videos" tab.)

In addition to the benefits of strengthening your feet and ankles, there is evidence coming from medical literature that shows that having our feet in contact with the earth transfers electrons to the body, in a process called earthing or grounding. It has been shown to reduce stress,[xlvii] decrease resting heart rate and even reduce red cell clumping in the bloodstream[xlviii]. I personally take time to go to the beach and walk in the sand each week to reconnect to the earth-mostly by playing beach volleyball! Plus, as you'll see in the Spiritual House, looking at the ocean is a great way to reduce stress too. The only catch with earthing is the surface you are walking on has to be made of "earth" materials, e.g. grass, sand, dirt or concrete. Concrete works because it's made from sand and gravel. Asphalt, used for roads, does not allow earthing as it's an insulator made from petroleum derivatives and stone. People ask me about floors in their homes. It depends what they are made of: the floor in my place is a composite, Pergo, made to look like wood. This is *not* useful for earthing (but of course it is good for the muscular training of my feet). Try earthing and see how you feel!

The Inner Environment

As mentioned before, environment is such a strong factor in our lives that a bad environment can overpower our good intentions and good habits. In most peoples' minds, by "environment" we would usually consider as a place, e.g., where we work, a bar, or nature. Over the years though, I have found that this environment, although important, is secondary to the environment in our bodies: namely our minds, feelings and spirit. Is it not true that these three things we carry around with us throughout our lives? It is of paramount importance that we look at the inner environment and get very clear about what is residing there and decide if we are ready to take steps at improving it.

PHYSICAL HOUSE WORKSHEET

Out of the following things discussed in the Physical House, which one do you feel you need to address the most? (Circle your answer below.)

Physical Activity/Exercise Sleep Eating Habits

What is one change you can make *today* in the area you need to address the most?

_____

_____

What stands in your way of making that change?

_____

_____

What can you do to remove that obstacle?

_____

_____

THE MENTAL HOUSE

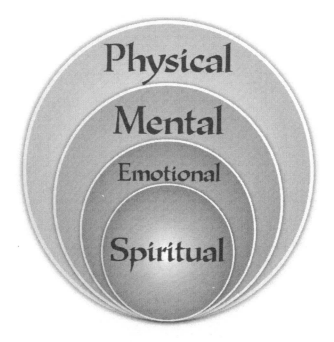

"Watch your thoughts; they become words. Watch your words; they become actions. Watch your actions; they become habit. Watch your habits; they become character. Watch your character; it becomes your destiny."

- Lao-Tzu

I have been interested in the field of psychology since I was an undergraduate at the University of Pennsylvania studying my major, the Biological Basis of Behavior. One requirement before we came as freshmen was to fill out a form which took a look into how we processed positive and negative life events. They asked questions like, "An event you cared about turned out really well. Was it due to something I did, or something completely out of my control?" Then you had to rate how much you felt it was "in or out of your control." It so happened that because of my answers on that form, I was pegged to be someone who was more prone to becoming depressed. I received a phone call asking me if I wanted to participate in a study, which at the time was called the Apex project. I said yes and was randomized into the study. I was either going to be in the control group, where no techniques were given, or in the study group, where we would learn some new cognitive behavioral techniques. I got a call and found that I would be enrolled in the study group. Through it, I was taught some cutting-edge techniques in analyzing my thoughts and how to change them to best benefit myself.

Of course, being 18-19 at the time, I really didn't like picking up an extra class nor having to fill out test forms, but I realize now, a lot of the successful thinking that happens now in my mind came from habits that were first introduced to me then. The biggest concept being that *my thoughts influenced my mood.* Moreover, *I could change those thoughts, and that would change my mood.*

If the literature on positive thinking and optimism has a father, it would be Dr. Martin Seligman, who not coincidentally was the lead researcher running the Apex project when I was at the University of Pennsylvania in the 1990's. I find this to be no coincidence as that experience *almost* led me to do a PhD and study psychology instead of medicine. Even though I didn't formally study it, I use positive thought on a day-to-day, moment-to-moment basis.

Looking back, it's pretty amazing how from that young age, I was given the tools in which to learn how to deal with my mind in such a way that it allowed me to be happy even when the world was not always giving me what I wanted (or at least what I thought I should have). Any steps along the way could have been missed: I could have not filled out that initial form, I could have not accepted the invitation to be part of the Apex project, and I could have been in the control group and not learned the techniques. That of course, didn't happen. I took that initial knowledge and over the next two decades began a deeper study of the mind and how it relates to our health.

The Importance of Mind-full-ness

The importance of mindfulness is that we finally get to see how full our minds are.

There's been a long-lost child running the show beneath our adult selves. Our minds are full of thoughts that are entrenched and harmful to us, taken as truth because they were said to us as children or because we agreed they were true. For mental health to really become a habit, we have to be aware of what we are allowing to enter the inner environment. We also must be aware of what thoughts are already there that have been overlooked that are potentially changeable. As we will explore in this section, there is a growing amount of data being "discovered"[2] showing the impact of our thoughts upon our physical health. This is why it is so important to really delve into the Mental House; it will allow us to rise to a higher plane of mental health.

The Words We Choose and the Stories We Tell

The words we choose to use are *so* important. Think about how we tell stories, how we interact, how we talk about events in our day. These things are important, way more important than the Western World gives them credit for. When we say or think things over and over, they become an affirmation, a statement that we make about ourselves, like a tape that plays automatically, *even if we don't want to say or think them.* (We will explore affirmations later in the Mental Section). The big point here is that you just don't want something that equates to a lower mental state hanging around longer than it needs to.

My favorite example is the difference between ex-plaining and complaining. Are we telling a story to simply

---

[2] **SIDEBAR:** Why did I put "discovered" in quotes? In our inexhaustible ingenuity, human beings feel pride when we think we literally pull something new out of thin air. As I learn more and more about the way the universe works, I realize that it's more that we *uncover* what is already there, rather than create something new. This is why I am always optimistic about every problem, because if it's a problem, that means that somewhere there is a solution, and it's up to us to find it.

relieve some of the pressure off the valve? Probably. But it goes much deeper than that. After beginning to tell a story where something bad happened to me, a little alarm goes off in me: *"Am I complaining? How have I tried to change the situation? How many times are you going to tell the same story?"*

We've probably all thought, "Oh no, here he/she goes again..." about someone close to us. An impulse in us rises up, wanting them to change, to get out of a pattern, to be happier. Turn that thought to yourself: When you're caught as the listener in that situation, frustrated, listening to a repeat story, STOP. Instead think to yourself, "how am I doing this exact same thing?" If you *never* noticed this about yourself, then it's time to become more aware, to consider the *possibility* that we might be doing the same because:

What we see in others, we have the seed of the same inside of ourselves.

Ever notice that when we are having a great day, everyone else seems to be happy? When we are having a bad day, cars are cutting us off and people are mean? If you have answered "yes" to this, the better questions then become:

1. Is this at all under our control?
2. How can we influence this state?
3. How do we create this state?

The truth is, we *can* control this reality, we *can* influence our internal state of mind and there are ways to do this. This is what the Mental House is all about.

The Terrorist

Part of the retraining of your mind has to be dealing with the voice of "The Terrorist." The Terrorist is that voice that consistently tells you that whatever you are experiencing *could* turn out bad. Or *is* bad. Or *will* turn out bad. Or has *always* turned out bad so why hope, why trust, why change, why heal? Everyone at some level has this voice trained into them, whether it is the internalized voice of a tough parent, or a voice that was created out of necessity because of unfortunate or abusive experiences in childhood. I call it the Terrorist because once you realize its presence you'll see that it strikes when you are least expecting, it hides in dark places in your mind, and it's been terrorizing you in the situations where you *should* feel the safest and loved. Our job, if this voice is getting in the way, is to A.) become aware of it, B.) decide to battle it, to challenge its "truths," because… well, they aren't true. It may feel daunting, especially when you realize how pervasive it is. Any chance you might want to take, whether big or small, you might hear that voice come up. The voice will be strongest when the issue is something near and dear to you. You might think that this voice would only stop you from big moves in your life, like quitting your job or asking for a raise. What I have found, where this voice hurts us the most, is when we choose not to speak up when our most intimate needs are not being met- whether it is asking for someone you love to do something different when it's been hurtful, or asking a partner to consider you first, when you have always put yourself last. What it really reveals on a deeper level is that we don't feel *worthy* of speaking up - because, as the Terrorist says, "Who are we to ask for such things?"

Make a list right now of things you have avoided saying, to whom, and then say why: (If the list is longer, pull out a sheet of paper and keep going!)

1. I'm avoiding saying _____

_____

to _____

because _____

_____

2. I'm avoiding saying _____

_____

to _____

because _____

_____

3. I'm avoiding saying _____

_____

to _____

because _____

_____

It is worth it to change, from a self-esteem standpoint, from a mental health standpoint, from a courage building standpoint, but the most practical reason to change is this: *The way that you have been doing things didn't work for your happiness.* So, the most reasonable thing is to try something new!

The Mental House Games

There's a lot of information in the Mental House section, some of which will help you become more aware of your mental habits just by reading it. However, I've noticed that what "sticks" often are The Mental House Games. This is, well, because games are fun!

Three notes about the games:
1. They are fun.

2. You play them with yourself. Or bring a friend into the game and compete.

3. Even if you lose, you win, because you learn something.

Game #1: Poise

Poise - (n.) 1. A state of balance or equilibrium. 2. A dignified, self-confident manner or bearing. 3. Steadiness.   (from Dictionary.com)

Objective: To maintain your poise around someone you usually do *not* have poise around, without becoming <u>worried</u>, <u>upset</u> or <u>angry</u>.

How to play: Choose someone from your life, who usually can make you worried, upset or angry. Before you enter their environment, decide you will play Poise. Choose a time limit and set a timer if possible. Look at your watch, mark the time, and say to yourself: "The Game starts now!" (And feel excited!)

Example: The friend at work who constantly is complaining about what he/she has to do, and constantly is talking behind people's backs about them, and is very draining to be around. You cannot *not* see this person because, well, you probably didn't hire them and unfortunately, he/she is the first person you see when walking in, and you have a habit of stopping to say hello. Before walking into the office, decide that "the Game starts now!" and do *whatever you need to do to keep your poise.* It may mean walking away, saying, "Sorry have things to do!" It may mean, passing by, just saying "Hello!" It may mean changing the subject a few times to something more positive. It doesn't matter, because the goal is to keep your poise.

How to win: Keep your poise for the allotted time.

How to lose: When you get worried, upset or angry.

How you win, even if you lose:

1. You are training your mind to remain calm using awareness and discipline.

2. You are finding out what situations trigger a loss of mental control. This is the main "win" as it really will allow you to see what stuff "gets you." If the "upset" is *way* out of proportion to the event (it sometimes is) then you have found what I call **mushrooming** of emotion. Mushrooming, which will be covered in the Emotional House, is the signal that there is undealt-with emotional energy present somewhere in your body.

When playing the game of Poise myself, I found that there were certain periods that made me more prone to becoming angry, upset or worried. For example, if I didn't sleep much the night before, that really affected my ability to stay "poised." Another reason was if I was overloaded in my schedule, and someone asked me to do something I didn't feel like I had the time to do.

If you try to have a friendly competition, it can lead to a really great conversation about why you lost Poise and what the other person does in that same situation. You might probably find that your friend also has the same issue sometimes, which makes it a lot easier to deal with because you're not alone.

Positive Versus Negative Thought

How many times have you heard that thinking positively helps? How many times have you thought, "Yes, that's true?" And how many times have you resolved to change your thinking but then kept on doing what you've always been doing: being negative when bad things happen? (For me, that would be a lot of times!)

I want to give you an explanation for this (to *partially* take us off the hook!) and also bring you hope. The reasons why it feels like an uphill slog to change your mind:

1. Negative thought is more powerful than positive thought when it comes to influencing behavior.

2. No one has taught us how to think positively, and *when* to think positively.

3. The world is set up to cue us to think negatively, from the news, from life situations, from the entertainment we choose to partake in.

4. Negative thought allows us to stay where we are. Humans don't like to change unless forced to.

Let's expand on this topic, go through some of the science, because it's very important to understand why we need to change our minds!

Flourishing Versus Languishing

Flourishing [xlix]is a state of being that incorporates optimal living in all ways, by thought, resiliency, growth and positivity. In simple terms flourishing means **thriving.** We all have experienced this state of being at one time or another, when it feels like "everything is going right," whether it's because we got a promotion, fell in love, made a lot of money or achieved something amazing. The problem is that for most people it comes as a result of something good going on *outside* of us. The real secret here is that feeling like life is worthwhile and amazing has almost *nothing* to do with what is going on outside of us. It has to do with how we *orient* to what is going on outside of ourselves. In other words, it's not what is going on around us, it's how we *think and process* what is going on. (Implied in this is that we have a *choice* in how we think and process.)

Languishing is the opposite end of the spectrum. It's a state of being in which things just don't seem to be going right, when sadness and "feeling stuck" predominate our awareness of our lives. Open up the dictionary and we find this:

>*to languish*: "to suffer from being forced to remain
>in an unpleasant place or situation."

We have at one time or another all felt this way and felt trapped and not able to get out of a negative situation. If we look back at those times, and ask, "how did we get out of that?", we'll immediately recognize the time and place where we decided to change. Ever ask a smoker (or yourself if you were one) "how they did it?" The answer is always the same, with some variation in wording: "I just decided to stop." The decision usually is stimulated by a realization, or a desire that is greater than us, like, "I want to be a better role model for my children." Thus, you have direct experience of what the scientific data shows, a direct experience of how the inner change precedes the outer change.

What is the key ingredient in making this dramatic and powerful change? *Willpower.* We suffered enough to finally awaken our willpower to make a decision to do things differently, to start thinking positively, to start thinking about how things can change. Then things did change.

What you will, when you are in tune with that Power, has to come to pass, because every thought that is given sufficient energy has to express itself. No causation goes without its effect.

Positive to Negative Thought Ratios

Corey Keyes and Barbara Fredrickson are regarded as the two researchers who pioneered these concepts of flourishing and languishing. The data has started to accumulate on how positive one must think to flourish.[1] They have described it in terms of a ratio of positive to negative thought. When giving talks, I have asked audiences what they think the average person's positive to negative thought ratio is, and most people guess that we think more negatively than positively. Surprisingly, it turns out that an average person (even one is who *not* flourishing) thinks more positive thoughts than negative, although in our day-to-day lives it may seem to be the opposite. An average person thinks at a ratio of 2.5:1 positive to negative thoughts. The reason why we seem to *feel* like we are more negative than that is because *negative thought is more impactful than positive thought*, meaning negative thought has more of a likelihood to influence our behavior, and lead to action or inaction, as the case usually is. So that's an average person's mind: 2.5 positive thoughts to 1 negative thought, and the result is, with that ratio, the person does not feel fulfilled. What's the ratio of a person who is feeling fulfilled, or flourishing? A flourishing person has a positive to negative thought ratio of greater than 4.5:1, meaning four and a half positives for every one negative.

How does one's thought ratio affect health? Well, a person who has a flourishing mindset has been shown to live a longer life, have less physical disease, and have less chronic illness. So, this is proof that the Mental House impacts the Physical House.

There are two important caveats to realize about this data:

1. No one thinks positively all the time. That's not the goal. That's perfectionism. The goal is to look to increase our number of positive thoughts and to avoid thinking negative thoughts. (We'll explore soon how to do this!)

2. No matter how long we have thought the way we have in the past, we can change our thoughts to change our lives.

Positive Thought and Immunity

As was presented in the introduction, cancer can be understood as an immune system failure. As presented in The Physical House section, anything that enhances the immune system's function and accuracy in detecting bad cells should be considered as an option to include. If you are like me and like to do everything that increases your chances of being healthy, you might feel excited to know that *how you think can improve your immune function.* Positive thought increases the function of your white cells, which are the foot soldiers of the immune system. Segerstrom et.al.[li] showed an increase in white cell count (specifically NK cells,

CD4 and CD8 cells) with mental positivity. This finding leads us right into an important emerging field in science called epigenetics.

Epigenetic Change and DNA Health

As you probably already know, DNA was discovered to be the "memory" that humans passed down from generation to generation, the information that allows us to look like our parents, walk like humans, etc. What was thought until recently was that DNA was inherited in a nonalterable fashion, meaning that what you got, you carried with you until it either randomly mutated into something different or you passed it on exactly as you received it (through your sperm or egg) to the next generation.

For the most part, this is true, you cannot change most of the DNA you have in you. However, a wrinkle in this understanding is epigenetics. Epigenetic change is change that occurs *outside* the DNA and also has the ability to be passed on to the next generation. The significance of this type of change is that it implies there are things that can influence the DNA and how it's expressed. The prefix "epi" literally means "above" and in this case, epi-genetic means that it is possible to *control what genes are expressed from outside the genes themselves.* Bruce Lipton, who is now famous in popular science for his work on epigenetics, has done a lot to shed light on this subject. In his book, *The Biology of Belief*,[lii] he goes into detail explaining that our thoughts influence our gene expression. If you have seen any popular motivational posters in friends' homes, you already know that this idea isn't new: *"Think and Grow Rich," "What you think you become,"* etc. What is new is that there is more and more hard scientific proof of this idea. For me, learning about this has been the tipping point where I finally said to myself: It's time to start embracing this concept.

DNA Health and Antidepressants

I was reading the New York Times a few years back and came upon some interesting research that really cemented for me the future of positive thought. A researcher, Owen Wolkowitz,[liii] had found a correlation between Major Depression and telomere length. The telomere is a part of the DNA structure involved in replication. It is generally accepted by researchers that the longer your telomere length is, the healthier your DNA is. In people who have had more episodes of Major Depression, it was found that those people had shorter telomeres. This finding has been replicated by other researchers[liv] as well, with a consistent finding that the more chronically one was depressed, the shorter their telomere length was.

Why are these findings significant? Researchers are thinking the shortened telomere is caused by stress but are not making it any more specific than that (at least at this point). The implication to me is that a negative internal environment- depression and by extension, the sadness and negative thought- was probably contributing to actual measurable damage to the DNA itself.[3] So, this is one piece of proof that the mind has an epigenetic influence on DNA. In follow up research, scientists have found that people who perceive events as threatening rather than challenging have higher stress levels (and consequently shorter telomeres)[lv].

SPIRITUAL HOUSE CROSSOVER: They also found that meditation practices can change the mind from perceiving things as threats to perceiving things as challenges, and also bring the mind more into balance. How is meditation working for these people? To put it simply, they are not barraging their internal environment with negative thoughts, adding stress to their internal environment. This is why in the above studies, the people who practiced meditative techniques recovered their telomere length- the DNA was allowed to repair: Meditation provides a concrete way to stop the negative thought so the *body can heal itself.* (We'll get more into meditation in the Spiritual House!)

Even before this cellular proof of the effect of negative thought and countering effects of meditation, there were the years of work done by cognitive behavioral psychologists like Dr. Seligman at the University of Pennsylvania. He demonstrated in multiple publications that challenging negative thought and replacing it with positive thought significantly helped depressed people become normal again.

---

[3] **SIDEBAR:** Scientists probably would say, you "can't prove causation" here. Just because it was "correlated" doesn't mean it's causative. This, thankfully, isn't a scientific journal. It's a book to help you heal.

In later research, perhaps even more significantly, Seligman found that replacing negative thought with positive allowed nondepressed people to thrive.[lvi]

I hope this section has provided at least some evidence that this "positive thinking stuff" as some of my skeptical friends might call it, actually is *real*. In fact, it is probably the most important thing you can actually change, and just as importantly, something you can change *right now*. As Lao Tzu, the author of the Tao Te Ching, said at the beginning of this section, "Watch your thoughts, they become your actions." One of my goals is to empower you, and not just empower you with hopeful ideas, but with effective tools that you can make your own and give you a sense of control over your health. "Watch your actions, they become habits." Breaking old habits of negative thought and victimization will be something you can control and take with you through your journey of healing and beyond.

"Am I on my side, or am I on my case?"
> - Mei Ling Moore, patient advocate

Stop the Chain Gang

You, me and everyone in this world has negative thoughts, but are they bad? Well, one thought isn't bad on its own. Repeating the same thought over and over? Yes, because as I said above, it becomes a habit to repeatedly think the same thing after similar events, and if the thought you have is negative, it will impact you for the future. (Conversely it can be a great habit to think a positive thought over and over!) Another subtlety: This section is about awareness of a thinking pattern I call "the Chain Gang." This is a gang of thoughts that link one after the other to drag you down, a mental fetter on your happiness.

When our minds are victimized, what happens to us when something bad happens? Or even worse, when something you *do* causes bad things to happen? We start to pour on the negativity, either directed at someone else ("How could she do this to me? Didn't they hear what I was saying? How could he be so dumb?") or directed at ourselves ("How could I be so stupid? Of course, this would happen to me! Why didn't I think of this before? If only I thought about this before. *Now* what's going to happen?"). Whether you are blaming someone else, or blaming yourself, there's only one person who gets hurt by this: ourselves. We have to learn to recognize this pattern of self-destructive and abusive behavior- and make no mistake- it's abusive. The opposite of this in Indian spirituality is called *ahimsa,* or the practice of non-injury. We in the West usually think of this concept of *ahimsa* as "do no harm." Moreover, we usually think of it in terms of hurting *others,* but on a deeper plane, *ahimsa* really means to stop hurting ourselves. (On a deeper level, hurting others *really* is hurting ourselves.)

The first negative thought isn't the issue. As I said, we *all* think negatively. The trick is to have the *awareness* to break the habit of the Chain Gang. Here is a game I created to change this habit.

Game #2: The OR Game

Objective: To come up with four or five positive thoughts about a specific event that you've already thought a negative thought about.

How to play the "OR"s:

1. A negative event occurs.

2. Become aware that you have thought a negative thought about the event.

3. Feel how "true" this feeling of negativity is. Rate it 0-100, a "0" being not true at all to "100" very true.

4. Come up with four or five positive thoughts *that are true* about the event as well.

5. Check in with how much better you feel. Rate it 0-100, "0" being not at all better, to "100" being completely better.

Time it takes: Should take under 3 minutes once you get the hang of it.

Example scenario: I'll take the easiest one we have all experienced: Someone you wanted to call you back does not call you back. You're upset, because it feels like the reason he/she hasn't called back is that he/she doesn't care about you. It feels 100% true that this is the reason. Four alternate thoughts: 1. He/she didn't get the message. 2. OR he/she hasn't been feeling well, and lots of calls have gotten backlogged. 3. OR his/her aunt got into an accident and they are very close. Everything else has dropped on the wayside while he/she has been helping out at the hospital. 4. OR he/she is bad at returning calls, no matter who the caller is. Rerate your feeling about not getting called back.

Why it works: This game is drawn directly from two pieces of research, from cognitive behavior therapy, which show that giving alternate explanations to yourself decreases the anxiety/distress and is protective against depression, and also using the 4.5:1 positive to negative thought ratio that was presented above. By experiencing the positives of a "negative" event, we challenge the reality that it's actually negative. We make it something that is beneficial, even if that benefit simply is putting forth the effort to try to be positive. The "OR" game starts a new habit, which leads to more profound changes over time.

Happiness Set Point

The effort we put forth in being positive has an additional effect on happiness. It changes your happiness set point.[lvii] What is a "happiness set point"? It is best defined as the habitual internal level that is comfortable to you to exist in emotionally and perspective wise, whether it be "really happy," "glass half full," "glass half empty," "waiting for the other shoe to drop," or "cynical." Your level of happiness is a habit, and you'll immediately recognize this pattern, if not in yourself, maybe in people close to you. Imagine someone who's mostly sad, who thinks of themselves as a victim in life. Their positive-to-negative thought ratio is about 1:1. When good things happen over a period of time (e.g. meeting a new love, getting a new job, having a great day, getting along with the family), the buildup of good events and good thoughts almost *cannot be tolerated.* Let me say it in a different way: The subconscious mind, because of its *habit* of "one positive to one negative" thought ratio, cannot tolerate this state of goodness, because it's not what it knows and is comfortable with. The subconscious searches for a way to reestablish its normal, so it creates situations or even interpretations of positive events in which to have negative thoughts. In this way, the comfortable, normal reality is reestablished. This is a sad habit, wouldn't you say? I myself had this habit in me for years, and the habit of cancelling out my positives was *immediate.* Example: I would get an acting job, and I would get excited, thinking, "I did it!" but then I would think, "Yeah, but it's only a few lines." Or, "Yeah, but it's not paying that much." Or any number of negative, defeating thoughts. The "Yeah buts" are a sign of this habitual low happiness set point.

The good news is that research has shown that you can change this set point. In fact, in response to major life stressors (cancer, anyone?), a good 25% of people change their happiness set point. Of course, this can be a change up or down. I would wager though because you are reading this book, the trend for you will be UP. Now that you are aware of the habit, you can use the following game to *build your positivity*, start a new habit and build energy to raise your happiness set point!

Game #3: The ANDs

Objective: To come up with four or five positive thoughts about a specific event that you've already thought a positive thought about, before a negative thought comes in.

Who should play: Anyone who knows they have a habit of the "Yeah buts." We are looking for "Yes, ands" !

How to play: Come up with five positive thoughts immediately after a positive event occurs.

Example: From my own life: I book an acting job. I think a positive thought, "Yeah! This is amazing!" Then I immediately come up with four more: 1. "AND I get to meet new industry professionals who get to see my work up close!" 2. AND "I will have people at the screening who haven't seen my work!" 3. "AND I get to be on set! I love being on set!" 4. "AND I will sharpen my skills in real on-set situations!" 5. "AND I get to add a line to my resume!"

How to win: You win by coming up with five *without* having a "Yeah but" pop into your mind. This is a fun game and you might be surprised at first how *hard* it actually is to come up with five positive thoughts in a row, especially without bringing yourself down.

How you win when you lose: If you notice that you have a resistance to even trying to play the game, you need to play it. It's not "stupid" or "silly" as your mind might say. If your mind does say either of these things, it's great because it will give you awareness of a cynicism you may be harboring from not allowing yourself to live in a state of happiness about something good.

> [P]rove me now herewith, saith the Lord of hosts, if I will not open you the windows of heaven and pour you out a blessing, that you shall not have room enough to receive it.
> -Malachi 3:10 (King James Version)

The Victim Mindset i.e., The Chronic Complainer

Part of taking ownership of your health is to stop complaining about the way it is. It's so enticing isn't it? It seems like complaining is going to make you feel better, to let people know how terrible life has been for you. (Please don't misunderstand: this is different than telling a loved one how much something they did or said hurts or telling a health professional what is bothering you.) What I am talking about is a victimized habit of thought, in situation after situation. Some examples: When the person in front of you in line gets a ticket and then you don't, because his was the last one; when a police officer pulls you over instead of the guy in front of you who was going just as fast; when something goes wrong at work, and it seems to keep happening to you. The basic thought is: "Why me?" or "Of course that would happen (to me)!"

What is victimization really? *Victimization is a deeply held pattern of thought that stems from low self-esteem.* The fact is, people who are healthy in their Mental House don't ask, "Why me?" all the time. They may feel frustrated at a situation, they may feel angry about a result, they may feel like something is unfair, but they never leave it at that. If you introspect on these situations, you might feel as if it is your *right* to feel upset at the unfairness of life. Of course, this is true, it is your right. However, is it what is best for you? Does it actually lead to happiness? OR does it simply justify what has already happened? Resolve to change your mind from victimized to victorious!

SPIRITUAL HOUSE CROSSOVER: These are classic examples of potential events that can be interpreted as "Why me?" types of events. If seen from a different perspective, these are *opportunities,* from a knowing down deep that *all things come to you for your growth,* even if it hurts, even if it seems unfair. Not only are they opportunities to practice positivity and seeing new options, but on a spiritual level, maybe it's for the best that this happened. However, this "blessing" or "good fortune" can only be received if the mind is open to the possibility of something good coming from something bad!

Game #4: Lemons to Lemonade

Objective: To create a new interpretation in unfair or unfortunate situations.

Who should play: People with a habit of saying, "Why me?" when seemingly unfair things happen to them.

How to play: When you feel a situation is unfair, or you got the short end of the stick, immediately look to find a way to make "lemonade" from lemons, or in other words, look for a "bright side" to the situation mentally. If you are resistant, recognize your thinking and at least try this expression: "Well, look at it this way, at least..." If you can do it before or soon after you entertain feelings of shame or upset or anger, then you have won the game!

Example: I am very avid Buffalo Bills football fan. If you know the history of this team, you'll know that this is a very easy situation in which one can go negative: Lots of strong feelings of connection, lots of identification, lots of desiring a good result, and unfortunately, lots and lots of bad results. Each season the Bills played, I had to find a way to turn lemonade from lemons, because, well, each season since I was young turned out to be a lemon!   Recently I went to a game and when the Bills started to lose in dramatic fashion, I could hear other fans saying, "Here we go again..." and "Of course..." and "Why, why, why ?!?!?" I started to think and say the same kinds of things, and I realized it feels comforting to jump on this "Victim Bandwagon."   After a minute of feeling this despair that was all around me, I turned to my cousin who was with me and said, "So glad we got to spend time together.   And it's a beautiful day to boot!"   This immediately made me feel better and I also got to let my cousin know how much I appreciated spending time with him. (To be completely honest, I still would rather have had the Bills win!!!)

The Use of Affirmations

"You will be a failure, until you impress the subconscious with the conviction you are a success. This is done by making an affirmation that 'clicks.'"
- Florence Scovel Shinn

As many topics in this book do, there is crossover to a different House. Affirmations are definitely one of these topics as they can be the bridge between the Mental House and the Spiritual House. We can think positively all we want, but if we do not *believe* the things we are saying, they are just words. If at some point, the body does not recognize, as Abraham Lincoln said, that "we hold these truths to be self-evident," then *the healing has not really gone to a level that will endure.*

An affirmation can simply be defined as a statement of truth. There are positive and negative affirmations. Any statement you say over and over can be called an affirmation. It's important to understand how to use them and understand their power. Throughout the ages, words have been used to shape the minds of others. Think of the impact of the word from powerful orators to create social change, whether it is for good, as in the case of Martin Luther King Jr., or bad, as in the case of Hitler. More to the point of this book, from India to Israel, healers have used the power of the word to heal the sick and infirmed- and we can use that same power to heal ourselves.

If you are laughing at this section and are ready to write it off already, you do run the risk of missing out on a powerful tool in your healing. In Asia, especially India, in Hinduism and Buddhism, affirmations have been used for thousands of years. A more familiar word that you may have heard is *mantra*. In fact, you've probably heard the phrase, "that's become my mantra" here in the West, but its significance has been diluted to a superficial meaning at best. In the Christian faith, the "Hail Mary" and "Our Father" are repeated over and over, as a form of prayer. These sacred prayers, when viewed from a different perspective, are healing affirmations. When I was a teenager, I went to Canisius High School in Buffalo, NY. Discipline was instilled using JUG, an acronym that stood for "Justice Under God." It was meant to be an inconvenience, a form of detention, which is common to many other schools. However, it differed in one particular aspect. We were forced to write a sentence: *"Promptness assists the learning process for all."* Unfortunately, it was never really understood by any of us serving JUG what this sentence really was. It was (you guessed it) an affirmation.

The "How to" of Affirmations

There are five keys to affirmations:

1. **Write them down.** That way you can repeat them and they can grow in power over time.

2. **Use only positive statements.** Avoid saying things like "I do not want a recurrence." "I am not sick." Write and say, "I am healthy."

3. **Use the present tense.** Do not say, "I *will be* healthy." or "I am *going to be* OK."

4. **Write and say sentences that are believable to you and increment them gradually**. If you are unable to say and believe "I am healthy," then start with something more believable: "I am getting healthier day by day." When that feels good, you can step up the intensity.

5. **Before repeating them, get yourself centered**, via relaxation or meditation, or deep breathing. THEN say the affirmation. Remember that tension is part of disease. (Remember: Dis-ease!) (We'll discuss meditation in the Spiritual House.)

Feel its power as you say the affirmation, its truth, and understand that you are *healing your body!*

One affirmation that I use when I teach my workshops to cancer patients is very simple and easy to remember:

I am whole and I am healed.

Please go ahead and make it your own!

People ask me, "How often should I be using affirmations?" I have gotten in the habit of giving it like a prescription: *10 repetitions, three times a day.* Of course, it's better to do more, but it's more important to get the habit engrained, because really, it's the *consistency* and *persistent* use, day after day that will affect a change in you. So, start with my prescription and continue it!

I have had my own doubts about this practice, as one can do them for weeks and months, and not see any tangible results. A senior and very wise monk named Brother Achalananda told a group of us once that he did a particular spiritual practice for seven years without a noticeable change. He began to get despondent about it, pessimistic about it changing. Then he decided to do something significant: He decided to keep going. One day he awoke to find that things had changed dramatically, overnight, with no particular reason on that day. It took him many years to figure it out, but he finally did. Being a former engineer before he was a monk, he used a science metaphor: "It's like an electron. Electrons live in orbits around a nucleus. To jump from one orbit to the next, you need a discrete (exact) amount of energy. Too little and you don't move from the old orbit, no matter how close to the number you get. Then one day you build up enough energy and BOOM, you leap up."

PRACTICAL NOTE: I use a calendar app on my phone and laptop to schedule out my days, and I put the current affirmation I'm working with "on repeat" at the same time each day, so I get reminded to say it. Try it!

SUCCESS NOTE: You might find that an affirmation that really resonated with you after a while starts to "lose its luster." It might be that you have grown, and it's time for a change to something different. Take this as a sign you are growing! Find a new affirmation in any area you want to improve to add to your mind!

Proof of the Power of the Mind

The "gold standard" in science is what is called the double-blind experiment, where one group gets the treatment and other gets the old standard treatment or a placebo. The providers are not supposed to know which test group gets what. The results then, are unbiased- meaning any hidden agenda a researcher may have, whether to demonstrate incredible results or poor results, are cancelled out. Thus, we can be more confident that the results are truly due to an effect of the experimental intervention whether it is a drug or a therapy.

In these tests, sometimes they use a placebo, or a "fake" drug to compare the experimental drug to. What is amazing is that they have found that those who took a placebo, 20-25% of the time, they actually *get better*, whether it was a decrease in pain or a lowering of blood pressure! Some researchers in ethics think it's unethical to give a placebo because it's not telling "the truth" to a patient, but some countries use placebos to treat people who don't need anything but demand something, which is really important in the case of antibiotic overuse. Putting that ethical issue aside, if you actually think about what the placebo effect is, it's a pretty striking piece of proof of the power of the mind. It shows us that the mental belief "This pill is going to make me better," actually really works to affect the Physical House! Conversely, there is a little-known effect called "nocebo" which in Latin means "I do harm," where patients receiving a placebo actually get *worse,* when they hold a belief that the pill they are taking is going to harm them. This effect can be up to 20-25% as well.[lviii] This shows us the powerful effect of our minds on our bodies.

Takeaways of the Mental House

1. Positive to negative thought ratio: To me, this is one of the most important aspects of mental health in disease *and* one in which vast improvements can be seen to be made in a short amount of time.

2. Positivity is part of health and it leads to improved immunity, healthier DNA and overall healing.

3. Using the Mental House games (Poise, The ORs, the ANDs and Lemons to Lemonade), we can make change FUN and, in the process, create new habits that will carry us through the rest of our lives.

4. Make affirmations a daily habit. They work, but don't take my word for it, try it!

MENTAL HOUSE WORKSHEET

Out of the following games and ideas discussed in the Mental House, which one do you feel will benefit you the most? (Circle your answer below.)

POISE   THE 'OR'S   THE 'AND'S   AFFIRMATIONS

What situations that are currently in your life can this game apply to?

_____

_____

Are you willing to try it the next time that situation arises?

_____

_____

What stands in your way of making that change? What can you do to remove that obstacle?

_____

_____

THE EMOTIONAL HOUSE

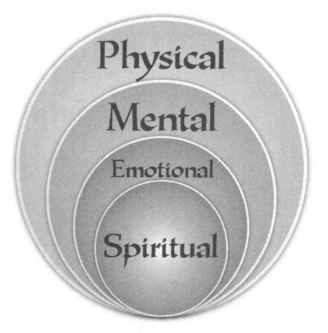

I find that most people on the road to health are very open to Physical House changes, especially nutritional advice. Some are even willing to address Mental House patterns and commit to a change. But, addressing the Emotional House? To find someone open to this type of work is unusual. I don't say this to blame anyone though, because our culture doesn't allow for emotional openness. It's more concerned with excess (reality TV), perfection (modeling and magazines) and political correctness (how dare you offend me!). In some cultures, this closed-off place is lauded as "toughness." You've heard it said in a tone of admiration: "Wow. I've never seen him cry."

Also, as human beings, we tend to shy away from the inside work, mostly because of fear. We are afraid to look inside at the pain and hurt that is there, afraid of the blame, shame and guilt we have harbored. I say this though: *To be aware of and to feel your feelings is a crucial factor in your long-term health.* Why is it so important? Let's explore this.

There is No Blame for The Past

Emotion is energy. Look at the word: *E-motion*: as in, *energy in motion.* If something awful happened to you in the past that caused you pain, especially on a repeated basis, the natural human reaction is to try to get away from it. If you were getting burned by a hot stove, you'd pull your hand away, right? Any sane adult would do this. But what happens if you can't pull your hand away? If you're forced to experience that pain over and over? *Your body would shut down, you'd pass out.*

Now imagine if you were a child, feeling this sort of pain, especially if it were coming from a parent. You'd have to do what you could to stop the pain. But you can't leave, because you need parents to survive. So, you do the one thing you can do: you wall off the pain and hurt – emotionally shut down- and keep on going, surviving the best way you can. Unfortunately, young children don't have the tools to take care of themselves, to set limits and boundaries and get their needs met, nor the mind to understand that even parents are human and all-too-fallible. As a helpless child, you have to believe that their hurtful actions *must be what love is* because if they aren't loving actions, it may mean that they don't love you (or even worse, that you're unlovable). Of course, this isn't true. It's just that true unconditional love is rare, and pretty much everyone has some wound from their parents, because parents are imperfect.

Even as an adult, this pain can remain trapped and reemerge in relationships where we play out the traumatic patterns over and over with current people who we attract based on these childhood traumas. It's totally understandable and totally confusing at the same time. Then, fortunately, we have children and unfortunately replay the same drama, but this time as the parent.

This phenomenon, known as transmission of trauma, is well known in psychology circles. If this description strikes a chord, and you recognize the pattern is present in your life, I encourage you to start this work now, to clear it from your relationships and your life. For your healing of disease though, there is an urgency to which I present the following section.

Emotions and Your DNA

Remember in the Mental House where we discussed the research about shortened telomere length and depression?

It has also been shown in additional research that traumatic events in childhood lead to shortened telomere length as adults, meaning again that the stress and toll of those experiences cause a lasting change in the victim's DNA[lix]. The takeaway from this is simply that those events do leave a scar. We have to do our best to heal those wounds, and not only will it heal our hearts, but our minds, our bodies and our genes.

Emotionally, Cancer is Trapped Pain and Resentment

Boom. There. I said it. Cancer can be, and oftentimes *is*, a physical manifestation of old pain and hurt, trapped in the body for a long enough time that it manifests in the Physical House.

This statement makes Western-only thinkers sit up, outraged: "What!? What medical school did you go to? What medical school did you learn this in?" The answer is that I didn't learn this in school. Instead, I learned from people who dedicate their lives to healing, from a different perspective: acupuncturists, herbalists, nutritionists, massage therapists, monks, energy healers, you name it. They all have said the same thing, in one way or another. After you hear the same truth spoken in so many ways by so many people who have dedicated their lives to healing others, it takes a really stubborn person to *not* listen. (DISCLAIMER:

It took me a while! Lots of the same mistakes, over and over.)

Remember:
"First God taps you. Then He pokes you.
Then He kicks you. Then he lets the world teach you."

These health providers definitely opened the door to a new understanding for me. However, the thing that turned me towards this as a real truth was doing something nowadays remarkable for a Western doctor: I listened to my patients. I listened as they talked about their lives. I began to see a pattern. After over 10 years of talking and asking specific questions about past trauma, I found that many of my patients were able to relate to me a story of high emotional trauma that had **not** been resolved in any meaningful way. This type of investigative inquiry is called *qualitative* research, which differs from *quantitative* research in that the former is more exploratory, looking for trends and patterns, and the latter is about numbers and statistics. This qualitative work can set up future quantitative research. (Interestingly, in medical school we only learn about quantitative research.)

Even though I knew what I was seeing was true, I was still searching for some "real" quantitative data, if only to quiet the voices in my head (and probably every critical Western doctor). I looked and looked but was unable to find anyone in the scientific literature who had looked at this question of trauma and cancer. I decided I would go ahead and keep writing my book without it, knowing it was a going to be a weak point. Finally, after I had written this section entirely, I was invited to a networking meeting of doctors and healers. I had a conflict in my schedule that I could not change, so I was going to skip it, but something inside me told me it was important that I go. I realized that I could only go for ten minutes with the drive time. It didn't make much sense to me, but I decided to follow my intuition. When I arrived, people were already there, talking before the official start of the meeting. One energetic doctor was talking to another person when that person excused herself. Without introducing himself, he turned and said to me, "Have you read the ACES studies?" I told him I hadn't. He said, "You must!" and walked off. I immediately wrote it down and soon after left the meeting.

I soon found out that ACES stood for the Adverse Childhood Experience Study, and it was exactly the thing I was looking for. The impact of the research is dramatic, unarguably valid and without question confirms the things I've discussed above. The study was originally done by Dr. Felitti and his team at Kaiser Permanente and involved over 17,000 patients.[lx] The methodology was rigorous and has spawned dozens of studies that validated the original study's findings, which were that adverse childhood experiences (including sexual, physical, mental, emotional abuse/neglect) contribute to and increase the likelihood of cancer,[lxi] diabetes, heart attacks, suicide, depression, and much more. It even used a 10-point questionnaire that is very similar to the one I had already written without knowing the ACE Study!

The other question I had was whether more recent trauma (not childhood) could affect one's susceptibility to cancer. I had heard quite often in interviewing patients that their cancer had revealed itself soon after a negative life-altering event like a spouse's death, or a parent's devastating illness where they were the caretaker. Indeed, upon searching, I did find studies that demonstrate that recent emotional trauma (divorce, death of husband or death of close relative) can lead to a higher risk of breast cancer.[lxii] I think that future research will be more definitive in looking at this question, if non-biological causes of cancer ever become a priority in Western Medicine.

Clinical story: Oftentimes as a last resort, people will bring their loved ones with an aggressive form of cancer to me to see if there is "something else" that can be done. "I want you to talk to Dr.V, he knows about this alternative stuff." My friend brought his father with advanced prostate cancer to see me, after he had gone through the standard treatments of radiation, hormones, and chemotherapy. His cancer had not stopped progressing, and his PSA values (used to measure cancer progression) were skyrocketing. He described to me his incredible affinity for what I was promoting, as he described it, "the combination of Western and Eastern science" in the fight against cancer. He detailed to me that he was following my advice to a "T," even before meeting me: He had for years adopted a vegan diet (no meat, no dairy), had been growing his own vegetables in an organic garden, exercised every day, slept without an alarm clock and finally, had been meditating (the cornerstone of the Spiritual House, as we'll discuss) for years as part of his health routine. Plus, he was retired, so his stress level was low and he was blessed because money wasn't an issue. For most doctors, this was as complete an approach as could be asked for. To be clear, I was very impressed. However, one fact remained. The cancer was still growing. Things weren't getting better.

So, I ventured to ask one question: "How is your relationship with your parents?"

His reply: "Everything is fine! I stopped speaking to my mother when I was five, and my father and I never really got along even though we lived together. So it's good."

I asked him if it bothered him that he didn't have any sort of relationship with his parents. "No. I just look forward, not back." Then I asked how his relationship with his family currently was. "Good, good!"

At this point, his wife burst out crying. "That's not true! You don't speak to your older son at all, and your other son, you (two) fight all the time." It was clear, after several more minutes that his relationship with his children was a mirror image of his relationship with his parents, a classic transmission of trauma. He finally admitted that he could see this was true, and the damage it had caused was obvious. Tears began to flow on his cheeks, probably for the first time in a long time.

"Have you ever thought about going to counseling or therapy? Seeing someone to help with your feelings?" He replied that he didn't believe in it but would "consider trying to go" because I suggested it. I explained to him how I strongly felt in his case that this emotional trauma was related to his cancer. I told him that looking at this issue may not change the course of his disease, but it was worth the effort to look, especially since he was doing everything else. We shook hands, he thanked me wholeheartedly and I offered to meet again in a couple months if he wanted.

At a follow-up call with his son, I found out he refused to go to see a counselor, nor did he wish to pursue anything further on the emotional front. He did, however, expand his garden, and wanted me to know that.

Clinical story takeaway: I shared this story because it illustrates several things, the most important being that this Emotional House work can feel very scary. It is very hard to consider looking at something very painful. To actually be courageous enough to say, "Yes, I see the problem and it needs to change," is brave in itself. Then to agree to step into the unknown, and then actually go out and *change*, it takes a lot of bravery.

Most of the energy is in the "getting ready to change," not in the changing itself.

- Craig Marshall,
public speaker & consultant

Yet change *is* what must happen. Let's dissect the above story: As a child without tools to handle loss, the man in the story above must have had severe emotional pain from losing the two primary relationships in his life. The fact that he was not mentally aware of this when speaking about it showed how blocked off it was from his experience. Even though he had done so many other positive things- nutritional changes, mental positivity, even meditation- the one thing that was most unhealthy he refused to address. The fact that it wasn't understood that it could be a source of disease is one of the main points of the Emotional House. Hopefully this helps to bring to life how emotional healing is a huge part of the story.

Even if you don't agree with this premise from a mental point of view, you'll have to see it from this point of view: The man in the above story had been doing *everything else.* He had exhausted all of Western medicine, been eating very healthy, meditating, thinking positively and had decreased stress in his life though retirement. The *only area left* that had not been explored (punctuated by his wife's emotional response) was the Emotional House.

If you want to look at it visually, let's go back to the visual "Houses" presented in the beginning of the book:

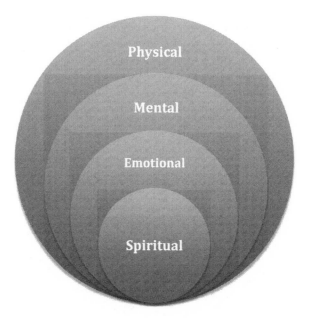

As you can see, all the circles are whole, relatively symmetric with the others.

In this man's understanding, his view of health looked more like this:

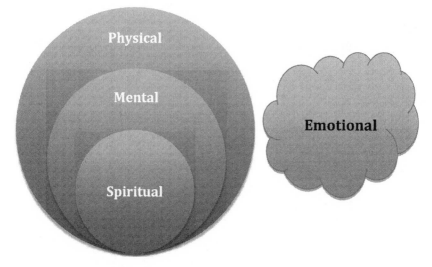

He thought, or at least unconsciously had accepted, that the Emotional House was totally separate. But in reality, this is what really is happening:

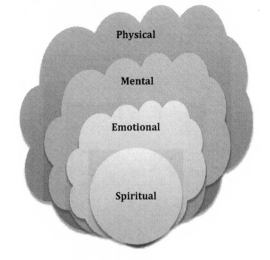

The long-held blockage to looking at the Emotional House had so affected his perception that he could not see that it was damaging the Mental and Physical Houses of his life. Okay: Say you are convinced, and say you agree with me, that this emotional trauma was a potential cause of his cancer's continued progression. The million-dollar question still remains: If it was a factor in his continued progression, and he were to entertain opening that door, i.e. starting to address the Emotional House, *would he heal?* Would his cancer go into remission?

This is a great question.

Of course, as with any great question, the answer is not so simple. The truth is, doing this work goes a long way towards real healing and *real healing is not about the body,* it's about a deeper level of peace and sense of well-being. This assumes that one has all the guidance and knowledge currently available, the courage and bravery to walk that path, and it also assumes that one has enough time to do that work inside to transform. Whether or not it "works" in affecting a cure is *almost* a side benefit to doing this work. I cannot tell you how inspiring it is to see patients who have already chosen to do this work when getting diagnosed, using it as a wakeup call to going deeper into themselves. One patient said to me, "You probably have never heard this, but I'm actually glad I got lung cancer. I didn't know my kids. I didn't know how to be happy. I just knew how to work. Now I know that I want to wake up and enjoy every single moment."

Whatever your belief about your past, it cannot hurt to take a look at it. Well, it may hurt to take a look at it, but I guarantee that the amount of energy and suffering one goes through from keeping that wall up, from the loss of relationships, of personal peace, of happiness and if you believe it, of physical health, far outweighs the hurt you may feel from looking at the Emotional House. If you haven't opened this door before, then this is a good time!

Questions that Need Clear Answers

I designed this section of the book to be more hands on, allowing you to be more introspective. Here are some questions for you to answer and reflect on. Grab a pen and fill in the lines. If you need more space, pull out some paper and continue writing. You might discover your mind saying, "I'll do this later." *Do not go forward until you have written these answers to the best of your ability.*

1. How is your relationship with your father? (Describe it.)

_____

_____

_____

2. How was your relationship with your father growing up? (Relative to now?)

_____

_____

_____

3. How is your relationship with your mother? (Describe it.)

_____

_____

_____

4. How was your relationship with your mother growing up?

_____

_____

_____

5. Did you experience any abuse in your house growing up that you are aware of?

_____

_____

_____

6. Was there anything that was "normal" in your house that you didn't see anywhere else in other kids' houses? Things that maybe other kids didn't have to deal with? (E.g., parent as an alcoholic/addict, a divorce resulting in the family unit

being destroyed, seeing verbal, physical, mental, or emotional abuse of a parent by the other parent, or abuse of a sibling)

_____

_____

_____

7. Do you have intimate relationships? How are your intimate relationships now (father, mother, husband, wife, girlfriend, boyfriend)?

_____

_____

_____

8. If you notice dysfunction in your current relationships, does it resemble any relationship dynamic from your childhood?

_____

_____

_____

9. Did you lose a close relationship suddenly growing up? (E.g. A close friend's accidental death, sibling death, parent/uncle/aunt/grandparent who was like a parent passing away suddenly?)

_____

_____

_____

10. Have you lost someone in the recent past (10-15 years) and "have not had time to deal with it"? (Not necessarily a death, it may mean an abrupt end to a meaningful relationship.)

_____

_____

_____

Look at your answers above. The reason I am asking these questions is to allow you to see if there are any flags here where further exploration may reveal locked pain and hurt underneath. Stated in another way, these questions are probing for clues to possible unresolved emotional issues. To be clear: If you find something that sticks out at you, this book is not the *end* of the work that needs to be done in this area, rather, it's the beginning of the work. Here are possible flags:

Questions 1 & 2, 3 & 4: FATHER AND MOTHER

Like in the example in the previous section, if your relationship with your father or mother as a child was traumatic and is still unresolved, then you probably know that this needs work. The chance of it resulting in a physical illness is probably *less* actually, because you are aware of the issues and the pain is still present in the Emotional House. However, if you have known it's a problem this whole time and have not looked at it, or have *avoided it* consciously, it could still be contributing to disease, because an open wound requires a lot of energy to maintain a boundary around.

If your relationship with your parent is good now, but was poor when you were a child, the question really is: Have you fully come to grips with the losses you had to absorb as a child? From my own life, I spent a lot of time rationalizing to myself: "Well, it's good now so that must mean that I let go of the past. It couldn't be good now if I didn't resolve it somehow along the way." WRONG! If you haven't chosen to heal it, then it's still there in some form. Just because things are harmonious now because you have changed the way you are dealing with said parent, then that means you've *adapted*, not healed. If your parent is the same and has not done work on their own to realize the wrongs committed, has not apologized and "made things right" with you (accompanied by your grieving of that loss), then it's *you* who has adapted to the "hot stove" and changed the way you've been around them to protect yourself. You've mentally *accepted* the situation as an adult. You've distanced yourself from that childhood trauma. The *lack of mourning of a loss* is a sure sign that there is unresolved emotional trauma underneath. The inner child is still angry and hurt.

Questions 4, 5, and 6: Childhood abuse and the abnormal home environment

I see this often: *Abuse at a distance of time doesn't seem so bad to the person who lived through it.* After all, you made it through, right? You have a family of your own now, so how bad could it have been? The reality is that humans have a tremendous capacity to survive. From a biological perspective, a human's goal is getting the body through emotional, mental, physical trauma so it can pass on its genetic information to make it to the next generation. Emotional trauma as an adult is easier to spot: For example, soldiers who become war veterans, we see emotional trauma show up as a syndrome known as PTSD (Post Traumatic Stress Disorder). It's easier to recognize because these adults cannot function in daily life and cannot take care of themselves. This shows up very clearly as substance abuse, homelessness, and depression. However, as a child, it's not so easy to recognize. The daily needs of a child are not provided by the child, rather they are provided by the parent. It may show up concretely as poor performance in school, fighting with peers or an inability to make friends, or something indirect like that, but in the end, the child generally *does not have the skills* to make his pain and needs known in a way that is clear to the people around them. *The strongest instinct in humans is to survive, not to feel.* If the child is adaptable, he/she finds a way to wall it off, and proceed through life, creating spaces around areas that are "not to be touched." Abuse can also come as neglect even. (See "The Mushroom Cloud" section underneath for a more in-depth discussion of this.) The obvious forms of abuse also apply here: sexual molestation, physical abuse, and mental abuse.

Questions 7 and 8: Current relationships

The trauma that lies in the answers to question 7 and 8 are more insidious. Take divorce for example. 32% of all American marriages end in divorce[lxiii] within 10 years. The "50% rate of divorce" isn't really accurate for this because 50% is a 20-year figure, and we are concerned with the first ten years of life where emotional trauma has been shown to be most damaging.[lxiv] This means a.) it's common and b.) it becomes accepted as normal because it happens so much. However, it's not normal. Not at all. Especially for the child of divorce. Many times, I hear, "My parents fought a lot so it's better they separated." This may be true, and it also may be true that it's a rationalization. Just because "we were better off" does not mean it wasn't painful to go through. After twenty or thirty years, it may be just a "fact" that your parents are divorced. However, to the child inside, it can still be a painful reality. It can manifest in the statement, "I never want to have kids." It may manifest in an inability to allow anyone to get close to you. If this is you, and you know that you have unresolved emotional trauma from it, it will pay to go deeper to heal this area. The second area I see people "think it's normal" is being the child of an addict, whether it be drugs, alcohol. Yes, it was normal for *you* but if you haven't dealt with it head-on via therapy or group therapies like Al-Anon, then it's probably showing up in your life symptomatically in your behavior: codependent behaviors, caretaking, a lack of boundaries, or even simply, and tragically, an inability to feel love. The clearest sign is your intimate partner having the same addiction as your parent did.

Questions 9 and 10: Death in childhood and adulthood

I have seen more than a few times patients in the cancer clinic who have experienced an unusual amount of death in their personal circle. One friend lost his father, mother, and brother *in one year*, in addition to his marriage and house. Two years later, he developed a hard to define blood disorder that was not really classifiable but very debilitating. It's so important to know that these types of losses, although part of life, can certainly affect your immune system and allow for disease to manifest.

Takeaways from These Ten Questions

I can't stress this enough: Fixing the physical manifestation of emotionally caused trauma only takes care of the problem temporarily. Maybe that's all you are able to do. I once had a patient who was in radiation treatment for her third cancer in twenty years. She said to me with resignation, "I'm here to cure the third one, so I can get the fourth one (that I haven't gotten yet)." She had tremendous unresolved issues, primarily with always being in her words, "the one in the family that has to fix everything because no one else can do it." At some point, the understanding has to come though that we have to put ourselves first. If we don't, then the ones we love that need our help won't get it, because we won't be there to give it.

How to Deal with The Past

Since we probably just unearthed a significant amount of old trauma, it's a good idea to **pull out a separate sheet of paper** and register what your mind is saying to you. We've taken a look at what emotionally driven issues may have impacted your healing, and your mind already may be clicking in: "We don't have the money to do therapy!" "I'm already tired from all the other treatments I've had to do." "This stuff doesn't really matter." I could sit here and challenge every thought you have, but guess what? You can too! You can challenge those thoughts, with the tools we talked about in the Mental House. (for example, the game The ORs!)

When dealing with the Emotional House, know this: *The untrained mind will not be your friend*. Or rather, the mind that brought you to this point will not be your friend. It's a collection of habitual thoughts that steer you to being *safe*. Safety is a great thing when we are talking about bears and tigers, but it's a detriment when it comes to internal work, especially changing long held patterns.

I am speaking from experience here. When someone would challenge me with new information about myself that was threatening, my first habit was always to turn it back on him or her: "ME?! What about you!? You do the exact same thing!" Then I would give them a few examples of how I was correct and they were wrong. Factual examples but only included to make my point: It's YOU, not me, that needed to change. The person speaking to me would- in a healthier fashion ironically- actually take a look inside and see what I was saying was true. But it didn't change the fact that the *reason* I was pointing it out was to defend my vulnerabilities and imperfections. It took me years to actually take a look at the pattern of defense I was using: intellectualization.

"There is nothing noble in being superior to your fellow man; true nobility is being superior to your former self."

> - Ernest Hemingway, writer

True change comes when you have a *desire* to grow, to be a better version of yourself, as Hemingway said. First you have to admit that you need to change. That can be a process in itself. For those of you with older parents, I am sure you hear this when you tell them they need to do something different in order to be healthier: "I'm too old to change. I am the way that I am."

That's just a false statement. You're *never* the same, from moment-to-moment, you change, and all the things around you change too. Mentally, you may keep the same patterns of thinking, but even look at the body: if this statement were true, would you get older? No. You'd stay the same. But you *do* change, you do get older, and with that, if you allow it, wisdom comes as well.

"You're either growing or you're dying.
So, get in motion and grow!"

> -Lou Holtz,
> football coach

Avoidance

When it comes time to actually do something different, this is what usually happens: We find something else to do first. We pick up the phone, call someone, clean the house, check the email, and watch TV- pretty much anything to avoid a positive action. Why? Why? Why? Of course, we feel regret and guilt later. But why? Why do we stop ourselves from doing something good? The reason we avoid is because there is *anxiety and fear* in the moment. So, we choose something pleasurable (or anything else!) to do instead. Take heart, because this is normal human behavior. Fortunately, this book isn't about doing what's normal, because as I said before, 'normal' is what got us here in the first place.

And as you know, "doing it later" a.k.a. procrastination, isn't just about our health. It affects everything- our dreams, our fix-it projects, our to-do lists- *everything*.

So how do we short-circuit this insidiously destructive pattern? This is where this next game comes in.

Game #5: Call of the Wild

Objective: To verbally call yourself out for what is going on in your mind

When to play: Anytime you are stuck or avoiding something

How to play:

1. As soon as you realize you're stuck or avoiding, say *out loud* what is going on: "I'm avoiding _____."

2. Then ask "Why?"

3. Say why *out loud*. "I'm scared it won't be any good." "I'm anxious that I'll make a mistake."

4. Then give yourself reassurance and say what you are going to do about it. "I know we're scared/anxious. That's ok. Let's do it anyway."

How it works: By saying the fear out loud, it makes a fear or anxiety less of an unconscious roadblock. It becomes less unwieldy and you begin to realize, *"Hey, this is just a feeling."* Part of moving forward is simply letting things come out and be what they are. A lot of what stops us is the fear of the unknown. This game attempts to remove that fear. Part of healing is letting what is real *be okay.* Try it!

Mushrooming

Mushrooming - (noun) when an emotional reaction to an event is much larger than what the event should normally cause if looked at objectively. Mushrooming signifies that there is blocked emotion in the Emotional

House that has not been looked at or brought to the surface.

What happens in a "mushroom" of emotion is that a minor event which is fairly innocuous (e.g. another driver cuts in front of you while you are driving in slow traffic, with no possibility of accident or injury) allows you to project onto the situation a blocked emotion. The sign of the mushroom is that the *amount* of emotion that comes up is *way* out of proportion to the event. It's qualitatively the same emotion (anger) but the *quantity* of emotion is much greater. Anyone who has acted out on his or her road rage (my hand is raised) knows how dangerous it can be to act out in an uncontrolled way. It can cause at best, emotional injury to oneself and at worst, physical injury and potential legal consequences.

So, you're asking, "Who cares? Who cares if I have road rage? Isn't it better to get it out?" To me, this is like letting the cover off a pot of boiling water instead of turning off the stove. You'll keep doing it, discharging your emotion but it never really solves the problem. It is better for your long-term health to address the *real* cause of the mushroom, rather than vent/blow up/act out in a seemingly random fashion.

This seemingly random event is called a *trigger*. Using the road rage example above, the anger trigger came from fear, precipitated by being cut off by the other car. ("That driver is an a$#hole !! What the f$%k is he/she thinking?")

193

If this is really taken apart emotionally, usually it opens up to something more personal: *not being seen/ not being taken care of.* In each person's case, the specific incident or incidents that caused this buildup of emotions will be different (e.g. mother not being there for you, being ignored during the parents' divorce, father shouting down your opinion as a child, spouse not taking your views/wants seriously) but thankfully the way to make it better is the same: If you recognize you are mushrooming as a pattern in your life, then the way to get clear is to recognize the initial trigger, to *feel those emotions* in a separate setting, then train yourself to be calm in the current situation.

For me, it has been a frustrating and enlightening journey to try to figure out a way to do just that: To feel what I feel in a safe way. In trying to navigate this world, sometimes we do things to simply survive. One of these things we do emotionally is wall-off emotion, or in psychological terms, we *compartmentalize* emotion. Why would we do that? To not feel out of control, to protect us from the *pain* that is felt when those emotions come up. This avoidance of pain is a primary driving force in life.

Now imagine yourself as a little child, not being able to care for yourself, and having a parent or relative hurt you over and over, emotionally. Since you're a child, there's not much in terms of *skills* in which to take care of yourself- you can't even leave of your own free will. So you're forced with a choice: either leave the family (impossible as a child) or numb yourself and compartmentalize the emotion.

Emotional childhood trauma (which can result in the formation of complex PTSD, a newly recognized form of PTSD from repeated psychological trauma[lxv]) doesn't have to be from parents who were drug abusers or alcoholics; it can be from parents who were otherwise very loving and providing. This can be hard to accept because no one wants to think of his or her parents as abusive. It doesn't mean that the parent or parents didn't do their best. We're just talking realities, facts, that may be uncomfortable at best and painful at worst. What kind of behaviors are we talking about? Calling a child "stupid" over and over (verbal assault), refusing to look at or touch a child (ignoring), not allowing a child to have friends (isolating), are just a few of these things. (For more, Google "Emotional child abuse" and it will list webpages that give a list of abusive patterns.) Chances are if you experienced these types of emotional trauma as a child, it's going to feel a bit disorienting to look at these patterns this way, especially if your relationship with your parent has become healthier. You might even be getting angry right now that I am saying this about them!

Some people and patients I talk to often are quite detached about their upbringing and very proud even. I had a friend who wore it like a badge: "My dad was pretty rough on me, slamming doors on my hand, and whatnot, but I think I turned out pretty well." ("Pretty well" meant strings of failed relationships and a workaholic existence.) Sometimes wearing the "White Coat" I hear these sorts of things but these issues cannot usually be tackled in a 30-

minute appointment about cancer. If the patient is open to it, I usually suggest that more work could be done in this area and if they want, I could refer them to an appropriate therapist.

Sometimes they laugh, sometimes they deflect, sometimes they accept the recommendation, but let me say this: When you leave in your wake a string of failed relationships (romantic or otherwise), are a smoker (and don't remember why you started) and are sitting in a clinic with a disease like cancer, there probably is a better way to go about how you handle that particular part of your past.

Realizing that as a child you did what was necessary to survive can remove a lot of the shame and guilt that comes along with this awareness. Know that whatever the situation was, from an alcoholic parent to an abusive parent, as a child or a young adult, you really didn't have a choice to stay where you were, and even if you did have a choice, you didn't have the tools in which to take care of yourself.

So maybe you see now, how that pattern has to change. The question remains, how do we take a look inside? Maybe we've had a recent blowup about something trivial and we realize now that it's not the real reason? This brings us to Game #6, one of the most valuable tools in this book.

Game #6: The Personal Inventory (or "How do I feel?")

Objective: To accurately describe and experience your feelings without judgment.

How to play:

1. **Go to a place where you can be alone.** Stand up. Shake off any nerves. (That gets you active.)

2. Say out loud to yourself, "How do I feel?"

3. Observe what is going on in your body. Are you tensing an area? Are you feeling tired? Sad? Are you worried?

4. When you have found something specific (it shouldn't take longer than 10 seconds), specify a **body** part or an **emotion.** Say, "I feel..." and use what word you feel, e.g. "I feel worried." If it comes with a physical sensation, say that too. "I feel worried. My neck is all tight."

5. Once you have said one thing, go right back and ask again, "How do I feel?"

6. Describe again how you feel. "My fists are balled up. I'm angry."

7. Keep going back and back, over and over, with whatever comes up. The game ends when you've run out of things to say.

Notes on how to play:

1. Examples of acceptable phrases: "I feel worried." "I feel tense in my neck."

2. You can use descriptive words to expand on your bodily sensations. "I feel angry. My hands are balled up and my jaw is super tight."

3. What not to say: "I feel **like** I am angry." Do not use the words "feel like." This is avoiding the real statement of "I feel angry."

4. Be careful of starting the sentence, "I feel…" and pausing and scanning, then saying "…angry." **Scan first** then say the complete sentence, "I feel angry." This allows a more definitive experience.

5. Do not analyze 'the why' of how you feel, for example, "I feel angry because I think that my brother shouldn't have said what he said to me, it's not right…"

6. The answers do not have to make sense or be related with the statements before. There is a natural zigzag to the game. "I feel stupid" and "I feel happy" can come right after each other. It's not a logical game, it's a FEELING game.

7. Feelings include **both** emotions and bodily sensations.

How and why it works for healing:

My acting coach, Kate McGregor-Stewart, a wonderfully spiritual and amazing teacher of life and acting, taught me this game. She has graciously allowed me to use it here. We use it to help access our feelings to become a better conveyor of emotion and behavior. What I immediately realized is that I felt more connected and *healthier*.

It works because it allows us a framework to feel things that are already there but are covered up by habits or societal norms. As you practice this exercise, layers of physical sensations are made conscious and thus allowing a pathway to get to deeper "blocked" emotions. The more one practices it and *allows* the body to respond the more healing will be taking place.

When to do it:

At least once a week. Specific times are:

1. Every time you are angry or disconnected. Every time you have an emotion that you've decided "isn't right to have." Let yourself have it!

2. Can be done in the car, when you are alone. (You won't be standing of course!)

3. Can be done with a friend, who can "observe" and let you know when you are not saying, "I feel" or are analyzing or are pausing between "I feel…" and the feeling.

Vulnerability

The feeling state you are left with after playing "How do I feel?" effectively is a state of vulnerability. This is the goal, the promised land of emotional health where the unknown becomes your friend and you can really start to feel fulfilled and healthy emotionally. In relationships, therapists often talk about "being vulnerable with our partners" which is excellent, but in the case of healing, it's not a vulnerability with others first, *but with ourselves* that really matters. Again, the mind here sometimes is not our friend:

"This is stupid."

"I don't want to be weak."

"If people see me doing this, they will judge me and think I'm a loser."

"If I fall apart from this, I'll never be able to put myself back together."

If there is a lack of vulnerability, what you might be feeling a lot of the time is 'I am alone.' This experience of loneliness is so prevalent in our increasingly isolated society that the means we use to cover it up are plentiful: Workaholic hours, excessive television watching, compulsive internet use, excessive social media checking, texting when we get just one free minute, phone calls when you are alone for a few minutes... you tell me what your escape of choice from loneliness is. There are a lot of great books and teachers that can expand on this topic but be careful!!! Figuring things out mentally or intellectually does NOT help you heal. You must express those feelings, release the old emotion. *That* is what helps you heal and find a vulnerable, healthy state.

What If I Just Don't Feel Anything?

Of course, some of you may be reading this and be saying to yourself, "What the heck is he talking about? Yes, I have cancer, yes, my mom/dad was mean or abusive or whatever you call it, BUT I don't really have strong feelings about it. Never have. It is what it is. Moving on."

That's okay, if it's not something you want to explore. There are a lot of other ways to approach health, and they are detailed in other parts of this book. However, there's a catch: Emotions are part of the human experience. You *do not have a choice* to have emotions or not. It's a part of human existence. I am not saying you do not have a choice in how you view something and react. In a segue to the Spiritual House: Yes, you have a choice in how you view an event. However, once that perspective is chosen, once you are engaged in a moment, "the choice" to have emotions is past. You're *in* the situation, and to be fully participating in a situation, you will experience emotions.

Let me be the first to tell you, I was a devout believer in "moving on" for many years. Whatever happened, whether a love relationship ending, huge parental disappointment, career failure, etc.- my way of getting through it was to say: "Moving on. 'No' Means Next!" This is a great business mantra, however, for personal failures, traumas and significant life changing events, this doesn't work in my experience. The problem is that "moving on" really means "moving on and bringing unresolved emotion with me."

After years of hardening yourself to pain and loss, you may feel like I have felt: *This is just the way I am.* Sure, I agree. It's the way you are, but the *real* question is, *is that way working?* Are you happy? Can you laugh, deep belly laughs? Is there joy? Or are you just walking through it numbly, "doing the best you can?" If you don't know where to start, maybe start here:

Game #7: Free Form Flow

Objective: To see what's in you, without judgment or analysis.

How to play:

1. Find a pile of scrap paper, more than you could possibly fill up in an hour.

2. Turn off your phone.

3. Go into a room where you can write for 30 minutes.

4. Start writing whatever comes up. You are not allowed to stop for 30 minutes.

5. Do not read what you wrote. Tear it up, throw it out, shred it.

Notes on how to play: You may find that you simply repeat one word over and over. You may find that you have nothing to say. Simply write, "I have nothing to say," or "This is stupid!!" Keep writing. Whatever comes into your head is what goes on the paper. Do not read it! This is not for analysis. This is for getting things out of your system.

How to win: By writing nonstop for 30 minutes. You'll find that things get unearthed!

Survival Over Feeling

Humans have an incredible ability to adapt to their circumstances. I have often thought about how proud I am about my ability to adapt, to "stay calm under pressure." However, what's missing is that we've been adapting not to an external circumstance, rather we've been adapting to life according to an unconscious decision we made long ago: *We chose survival over feeling.*

Sometimes, under extreme duress, we have to make quick and often lasting choices about how to cope. Sometimes we don't even know we are making choices at all. For a close personal example, my field, Radiation Oncology, is a special field. We interact with some of the most alive people in the world: cancer patients. They are alive because they know, finally and sometimes for the first time, that their lives aren't permanent. *They might die from this.* And that gives a burst of life like you wouldn't believe, noticeable to the patient and the doctor treating them.

On the other hand, 30% of our patients come with a diagnosis that is incurable. These patients die, oftentimes right within our care. As oncologists we are trained, yes, but not trained for this level of loss and emotion. The simple, brutal fact remains: It's not normal to see 30% of the people you meet die. So what happens? We say in our heads, "We did the best we could. Got to move on."

You know what *really* happens though? We become numb. Because we've blocked ourselves off from mourning, from experiencing the loss, because if we did cry over every patient, every person, we think we'd be a wreck. The reality is, many of my colleagues are wrecks because they *don't* feel what is going on. They either carry around so much locked emotion that they can't feel anything or they act out in some way to try to escape the emotional situation. They may attribute this to another reason entirely, but from what I've experienced, this choice of survival over feeling is a significant reason why.

The Seven Emotions

From my work in the field of acting, I've gotten pretty well versed in the emotions, because there are really only two things actors are providing: behavior and emotion. People ask me all the time why I love being an actor, and it's pretty simple. It has taught me so much in terms of being true to myself, feeling my own feelings and learning how to express those feelings. I have no doubt that without this training, I wouldn't be the man or doctor that I am today. One thing I have incorporated from my first acting coach, Joe Palese, is that I have to access to all the emotions. He used to teach that there are seven basic emotions, plus or minus one depending on where you read. This may come as a shock to you. Let's go through it and break them down. Can you come up with the seven? (Don't look to the next line because they're there!)

The seven are: Anger, Love, Joy, Sadness, Jealousy, Hate and Fear. [4] Every other feeling that we have is a variation on these seven and the colors and variations on these basic seven are endless. (Again, depending on where you go and look, there may be variations in what a scientist or acting coach calls an emotion, but let's not get derailed.)

For our purposes, the most important one to look at is anger. Anger manifests itself in many forms: frustration, resentment, rage, annoyance, and being pissed off. Whatever word fits your experience, they are simply different shades of anger put through the scope of your mind, with different intensities. Sometimes in trying to rationalize or deal with our anger, we will minimize it by choosing a word that doesn't exactly fit what is going on inside. (The most common is when we say, "that's annoying," when we really mean we are very angry.)

In cancer, the main culprit emotionally is resentment. If you take a look at what resentment really is, you can see that it is an anger that comes through a perspective of "It shouldn't have been this way." It lingers and is about something that happened in the past. It's a pretty *stuck* feeling, isn't it?

Here's the rub: *Resentment is NEVER the root emotion.* Once you admit that you are resentful, and start feeling it (say, by playing Game #6: The Personal Inventory/How Do I Feel?) you'll see that underneath the anger is hurt and

---

[4] Check this out: there are seven basic emotions, seven prime colors, seven major notes in music. Someone is up to something! And it's cool!

sadness. This is where the tears come out. Lots of people choose to turn off the path at this point. The feeling I have felt and have heard others describe is a sense that "if I feel this pain, it will be so painful that I'll die or that I won't be able to take it." This is a lie of the mind. The thing that one needs at this point is courage. If you are able to feel this anger as resentment, then feel this pain and sadness underneath, then guess what's underneath that? You. And Love.

Sometimes you have to dig up the dirt first to get to the gold buried underneath.

My point in bringing up the seven emotions is that we as humans are born with the ability to feel all emotions (unless you have a mental illness like sociopathic personality disorder). A lot of people I have met have an inability to access certain emotions. (Note that I used the word "access" and not "feel." We all have the ability to feel. We may not all have access.) When I first began having romantic relationships, I noticed I was having a hard time accessing love. For a long time, I thought, "That's just the way that I am," or "Maybe I am feeling it, and just don't know it." The reality was that there was a whole bunch of blocked emotion sequestered in my body, mostly sadness and resentment, that was covering up the feeling of love. Here's a fact though: If you can feel one emotion, you have the ability to feel them all. The catch is you must *want* to feel it. You can also alternatively choose to not feel it, but you will have to accept this fact: You will always know that there is *more,* deeper inside you, and that every time you have an experience, the experience will only be 80% of what it could be. You may never feel all the pain of an event, but you'll also never feel all the love of another. That's a choice that is up to you.

> *If in your fear you would seek only love's peace and love's pleasure,*
> *Then it is better for you that you cover your nakedness and pass out of love's threshing floor*
> *Into the seasonless world where you shall laugh, but not all of Your laughter, and weep, but not all of your tears.*

\- Khalil Gibran,
from the Prophet[lxvi]

Emotional Feelings and Intuitive Feelings

This is a crossover to the Spiritual House and is a subtle point, but something I think worth mentioning: In the West, we lump emotions and feelings into the same basket, and use the terms interchangeably. However, there are other perceptions that we also lump into feelings that originate from a deeper place, namely your intuition. These intuitive feelings, which are not emotions at all, act as guideposts for you to consider in any situation you are in. Examples of intuitive feelings are:

1. When you "know" someone is not good for you to be around, you may get a "feeling" that you cannot trust that person. You may still have to be around them by choice or circumstance, and when they eventually turn against you, you'll say, "I knew it from the beginning."

2. When you feel that someone is supposed to be a friend to you, you immediately start treating him or her like you've known them all your life. You "click" and you know it.

3. When you are working in a job, and it just feels "right." Alternatively, the job may tick off all the requirements you asked for, but it just never really makes you feel "at home."

I'm sure you can think of more 'intuitive feelings,' and it's good to have a sense that these are different from emotional feelings. These intuitive feelings do not change over time, nor do they need to be cleared out like emotional feelings. They are really a guidepost to you about what is right for you and what is not. How do you develop this further? We'll explore that in the Spiritual House.

Mourning Old Losses

Lots of times as children we don't have the ability to fully feel and process the incredible losses that happen to us. As adults we may be more "mature" but many times we are *still* unable to feel the impact of huge losses. As discussed before, these things pile up, and they come out as repeated patterns and mushroomed events that disconnect us from our lives. We think, "Let's just get past this," "Let's move on," basically thinking *anything* besides what will really heal us.

What is mourning really? Merriman-Webster dictionary defines it as, "to feel sorrow or grief for." Even before that sadness, one has to have the recognition and awareness that *the thing we lost was important to us.* It's a natural thing to mourn loss, but cultural training and familial training get in the way. Since childhood I have been fascinated by elephants (maybe because my family is from Thailand). Researchers have observed elephants coming from miles to be near the body of a deceased older elephant that was a leader in the community. (Google "elephants loss mourning" and you'll see a video on it). Now we don't have insight into what the elephants are thinking but many people believe they are mourning. It makes me think about how it's okay to cry over the death of a loved one, but for some reason this is the only acceptable thing to mourn in most cultures.

The fact is, there are things we lose that may arguably cause as much pain as the death of a loved one. Unfortunately, we may not feel comfortable displaying this grief in front of the ones we love or even the ones that are there when the loss occurs. We bury it, and sometimes we pretend it doesn't hurt us. What I am suggesting is that when we get to a safe space, it is *so* important to access the grief. Even more important: If we can get awareness of what this process looks like, then it's easier to let it happen and not get in the way.

What does mourning even look like? Well, let's look at the thoughts that come up; they are clues to what feelings lie beneath. The markers, originally identified by the researcher Elisabeth Kubler-Ross, have been identified as "stages" of grief: anger, denial, bargaining, depression and acceptance. I hesitate to use the word "stages" because it gives the impression that there are distinct, separate phases, where in reality it may flop from one to the other on any given day. This isn't a complete list and neither is it necessary for all five to occur for healing to take place. Each loss will have its own course. And again, it's not just about death and loss of a loved one.

Here are some losses that can fit the bill for a mourning process:

- Loss of a job you loved very much
- Loss of a house (through bankruptcy, fire, or natural disaster)

- Loss of a relationship
- Loss of the hope of having a relationship (father, mother, friend)
- Loss of a dreamed-about future due to personal disease
- Loss of a long-held childhood dream (especially when confronted by a stark reality)

Take the recent loss of an exciting job I had. Below are the thoughts that came up when the loss happened. Instead of saying, "That's OK, one door closes and another door opens," I let the feelings occur and gave myself an opportunity to feel the loss. After each thought I had, you'll see what stage of loss they might fit into:

"What? This can't happen to me?!"   (DENIAL)

"What did I do (to deserve this)?"   (ANGER)

"If I would have only (done that) this wouldn't have happened… maybe I could apologize..." (BARGAINING)

"What a $!%@%, how could he do this to me?" (ANGER)

"What am I going to do now?" (DEPRESSION)

"Maybe I can figure it out, maybe if I do this, I can save my job..." (BARGAINING)

"How come everyone gets what they want except me?" (DEPRESSION)

"I worked so hard to make it work..." (DEPRESSION)

"I was honest and he lied. Next time I won't trust anyone." (ANGER)

"It's okay. There will be more coming my way." (ACCEPTANCE)

I wanted to give you these specific thoughts to show you it's *normal and human* to have these thoughts. There wasn't much healthy modeling in my family to allow these thoughts to be "OK" in my head, and because of that, I suppressed a lot of grief from loss. If you have these thoughts when thinking about an old loss (from childhood, recent relationships), know that they are 1.) A signal to you there's loss/grief beneath them 2.) These thoughts are normal in the process of grieving. But *we* arrest this process. The only thing to do is to go back in there and feel them and process them using the tools we've discussed, especially The Personal Inventory and Free Form Flow. Even with these games, we may not be able to find our way in without help.

After you have given yourself a chance to feel the feelings, *then* it's okay to move into the "you'll get the next one!" phase. But don't allow yourself to be fooled. There was a loss. It may only take five minutes, or it may take five weeks, really the important part is to let yourself have the experience. (CAVEAT: If you have mourned a loss for a really long time and the feelings don't seem to be going away or seem to be getting worse- the American Psychiatric Association generally lists over six months- it would be in your best interest to contact a professional to help as it may be pathological rather than healthy mourning.)

Therapy Versus Antidepressants

Having a background in psychology, acting, and having gone through a formal therapeutic process myself, I am very quick to recognize when a cancer patient has a tremendous amount of emotional energy locked up in them. Oftentimes when one goes through a traumatic life-changing event like cancer, the adjustment itself to this news can become worthy of counseling (called in the DSM[lxvii], "Adjustment Disorder"). However, there is often a deeper layer, the one we have been describing above, where what has been long buried starts to surface with the change-in-life situation. In both of these cases, and when the patient is open to it, I refer the patient to a therapist. I don't presume to have the expertise nor the experience to tackle those issues that may take months or years to actually open up and heal, like abuse and strongly held patterns. One good thing is that nowadays, insurances are paying for this type of counseling, because of the well-documented fact that patients with cancer can often have mental side effects as well. (I hesitate to use the term "mental illness" due to its societal connotation as something terrible. For me, it's the same as physical illness, just of the mind but I know our society can have a prejudice against those labeled with "mental illness.")

Antidepressants (like Prozac [fluoxetine] or Effexor [venlafaxine]) can often be a "quick trigger" medication to get people through a tough adjustment period, especially if they are laden with a lot of life stressors that need to be dealt with. Providers often utilize medications to help people get over the hump and many times the patient requests them. I know a lot of patients who have been helped by these drugs, so I'm not against them in those situations.

My main concern with using them is that instead of being used as a way to get people through a tough period of months, patients never get off them and instead are on them for years instead of using them as a bridge to some real change. In other words, instead of helping patients heal and bridge a gap, antidepressants become a crutch for people to stay stuck. Again, in my opinion, they can be a great tool when given with the intention of a bridge to a change that is more durable and that comes from inside (i.e., pairing it with therapy and a therapist).

Psychodynamic-Based vs. Cognitive Behavioral Therapy

There is an academic "war" going on between these two types of approaches to psychology. Psychodynamic-based psychotherapy uses an approach that looks to bring awareness to a maladaptive pattern that has been at least partly unconscious in a person's life, usually from early childhood. Cognitive behavioral therapy on the other hand looks to change current thinking habits using practical tools and fixes, not looking to the past at all. Having personally experienced both ends of the spectrum in psychological treatment, cognitive behavioral therapy (CBT) and psychodynamic therapy, I can say that both were effective for me for different reasons. CBT is useful in a very practical way, to get our minds out of a distorted view of reality, to challenge what we are saying by confronting our minds with actual facts. For example: After realizing we have made a very bad mistake: "I'm so stupid." You would learn to challenge this: "Well, I finished college and graduated with honors. Also, people come to me all the time for advice. How stupid can I really be?" (Apologies to CBT therapists: This is over-simplified, but it's just for a quick understanding.) Psychodynamic processes look at long held beliefs and try to find their origins, usually finding the root in the parent-child stage of development. By relieving the guilt and hurt from these past experiences, the current maladaptive patterns are easier to understand and change.

I have experienced practitioners of both types and the truth is, experienced practitioners use both types of approaches either knowingly or unknowingly. The reason for this is that most psychologists genuinely want to help people, and if they feel something in their "bag of tricks" will apply to someone suffering right in front of them, they won't hesitate to use it.

If you look back to the Mental House, where I had you play the game of The Others, that game was from the files of Cognitive Behavioral therapy. When I asked in the Emotional House about your history of your past relationships, that was from the files of the psychodynamic model. So, you've been exposed to both and can see how both would and could be useful.

The question becomes, which one to choose? If you are mostly depressed from the new reality you have been placed into by the diagnosis, then Cognitive Behavioral therapy has been shown to be very effective in this case. The time course of CBT is also shorter, which financially and timewise is advantageous. The answers to the above parental relationship questions should give you some data as well. If you answered, "yes" to any of the parental/childhood questions, and feel there is unresolved emotional trauma lurking, then a psychodynamic approach is important to consider. This treatment is definitely more therapist specific (meaning you should go to a therapist who is highly recommended) and it also takes longer.

The thing that saddens me with people who actually have gone to psychodynamic psychotherapy with a trained therapist is that a large percentage (40-50% in some studies) quit before meaningful lasting change is made. Oftentimes there is a process I have observed, where it goes from "This therapist is great!" to "I don't think this is working..." to "I hate this guy!" to "I am really beginning to understand myself and why I have been doing what I do." Sadly, people seem to quit before the last stage occurs. Of course, you probably know people who have been doing the therapy process for years and do not seem any better. What is the optimal length? The data[lxviii] suggests that 50 weeks of treatment is a significant number for psychodynamic therapy. What I found encouraging is that the effect of the treatment lasts well beyond the end of therapy, meaning improvement is seen well *after* therapy has ended, even to a few years out, which to me means the therapy really worked.

How Do I Know That the Emotional House Actually Improves the Physical House?

The connection from the Emotional to the Physical is hard to quantify, primarily because most Western-trained scientists are not looking to make this connection in scientific literature. Of course, in the Eastern annals, which do not conform to Western standard of formal study, the evidence is overflowing. That being said, I did comb the Western literature looking for "proof." Dr. Allan Abbass has shown that short-term psychodynamic psychotherapy showed a highly significant decrease in physical symptoms if patients completed the therapy.[lxix] Symptoms like back pain, headaches, migraines, stomach pain, diarrhea- things that one would not ordinarily think would get better -- all improved with "emotional" treatment. This provides one piece of evidence that working on the emotions directly will actually improve your physical body.

Unfortunately, the "gold standard" of evidence, the double-blind experiment, has not (yet) been used for relating emotions to disease directly. This will probably come in time, once healers and doctors start to really become interested in the integration of healing. As I said earlier, for the Emotional House, a lot of what I have learned came from Eastern medicine practitioners and by asking patients. When I stated before that "emotionally, cancer is resentment," I came to that understanding by asking patients first hand. As you saw earlier, there are three questions that I ask: How was your relationship with your parents growing up? Did you experience any abuse growing up? Did you experience any emotional trauma? In over 90% of people, the answer to one of these questions is inevitably, "yes." Obviously, this is not a rigorous methodology by any means, but it convinced me enough to put it out there for you to digest. (Only later did the landmark ACES study, which showed a definite link between emotional trauma and cancer, pop into my consciousness.) This is new in the West as a concept, but no one with an Eastern medicine background would blink an eye if I said it. (I do feel more comfortable that 3,000 years of Eastern practice backs up my experience!)

The Role of Mirror Neurons

I've used the word "environment" throughout the book and now I want expand on it. There are two parts of the environment, your inner environment and the outer environment. One of them (the inner) is under your control to a great extent, with what you eat, how you think, and how you feel, all under a good amount of control. The other, the outer (external) environment, is often less under our control. We have oftentimes little control over who is working around us, who lives with us, or what jobs we have. Changing these things can often require a big "pivot" or game-changing decision. The secret is after doing a lot of the inner environmental healing, the outer environment often changes as well as a result. Sometimes I have seen it simply "happen" where someone loses a job only to get a much better situation fall right into their lap. Other times, the changes that need to happen on the outside becomes obvious, and to make them happen requires a conscious choice, but takes less effort because the momentum to change has already been established on the inside. Because of this knowledge, I have chosen to not spend a lot of time on the external environment in this book. That being said, the external environment does have a significant interplay with the emotional circuitry of our brains through the mirror neuron network.

A normal motor neuron fires in your body when you want to move a body part. For example, to move your right arm, a motor neuron in your left motor cortex would have fired first, then the arm would have moved as a result.

A *mirror* neuron is a specific type of motor neuron. It is peculiar, because it fires when you see *someone else* moving his or her arm. Why would that happen? Well, humans learn a lot of their behaviors through imitation. The mirror neuron is thought to be crucial to this process. If we can observe a fellow human doing something and incorporate it quickly, it serves to give the observer an advantage in life. Think of all the things we learn best by watching someone else do something!

What makes the existence of a mirror neuron more intriguing is that is also fires when you witness another person have an emotion. Researchers have shown that an observer's stress hormones go up when watching another person get yelled at, even if they don't know the person. It is even more interesting, because their stress hormones went up even if they would not have been upset if they were getting yelled at themselves! [lxx] What does this mean? This means that being around people who are angry or stressed out often causes *secondary stress* on the people in the environment. This is why it is so important that we choose our companions and our workplaces carefully, if possible. The research also shows that if you actually know the person getting yelled at, your stress levels go up four times higher than if you didn't know them. This explains also the effect fighting in the home has on family members, especially those most vulnerable: children.

Interestingly, the mirror neuron effect also happens when one is watching an event on television, but to a lesser degree. This is why TV is so sneakily damaging: we *think* we can watch things from the safety of our own homes, but in reality, it still can affect us in a harmful way if we are choosing to watch events of torture, death, war and conflict for "pleasure purposes." It may be an escape, but it's definitely not healthy.

Mirror Neurons: Empathy and Healing

The news isn't *all* bad, of course. You can feel not only stress from mirror neurons but love and peace as well from their effects. By choosing our environments, we can often cause an outer-to-inner change. Spending time around happy people at peaceful locations- community service projects, parks, churches, meditation centers, or just out in nature, for a few examples- these environments can affect internal healing just by putting yourself in them. You've already known this probably from experience, but now you know because of the mirror neuron network, you are allowing your brain to experience healing effects.

You may ask, what about people who are sad or depressed? Are we supposed to avoid these people? If someone is going through a tough time, of course, it pays to be supportive as long as you are consciously directing the flow of energy towards that person. This is different from being around someone who consistently is a victim. (You already know who I'm talking about in your life, don't you?) They are hard to be around and being around them and not getting sucked into their energy is a battle. A coach of mine, Barbara Deutsch,[5] compares personal relationships with being in a theater: Some people you want on the stage with you (to share your intimate details), some people you want in the audience (to witness but only so much), some people you want in the lobby (because they can't be trusted to keep you in mind). We each have to decide where people in our lives should be. I have come to understand it as such: *People belong where we can love them.* If we resent them or they hurt us by being on the stage, then we have to move them further out, into the audience, or the lobby, or sometimes totally out of the theater. Take a good look at who is in your life and do your best to be healthy with those relationships. Create boundaries. It's not depriving them of something good if all you do when together is fight. This especially goes for family members. We think that because they are family, they deserve to know everything and be on the stage. This is NOT true. Sometimes family members need to be in the lobby. Telling them they have "lost some privileges" may spur them to reconsider their behaviors, at least around you!

Considering the mirror neuron again, what does it mean that our brains "fire" when seeing another human going through a tough time? It means that our brains are hard-wired to be empathetic, i.e., to feel for someone else.

---

[5] Check her out at thebarbaradeutschapproach.com

For me it goes to this idea: *You cannot feel for others what you do not feel for yourself.* I have often talked to patients who feel that they cannot experience certain emotions like sadness but cry when they see sad movies or clips on YouTube. This means that if you can feel sadness for someone else's situation, that you must have, at some point, been able to have the same feelings for yourself. Again, a lot of people with cancer have great empathy for others, yet for themselves, they tend to minimize the effect of events on their lives and experience. Most of the time, there is a frank *denial* over the emotional impact.

I have noticed this in myself- I could get extraordinarily angry when someone was threatening a loved one, yet I strangely felt no anger when the *exact* same situation happened to me! Oftentimes a friend would need to point it out to me, "Hey doesn't that make you angry? That even pissed me off!" The same goes for sadness: I could feel sadness for a character on a movie screen, yet, for traumatic events in my life, I couldn't feel a thing. If this happens to you, it's a good sign that there is a profound disconnection or in psychological terms, a disassociation. Just as important, there is a blockage in emotional release. Remember: e-motion is energy in motion! For most people suffering with disease, this emotion is not "in motion." It's stuck. And most of the time, we don't even know it. I used to think that because we have trauma, we develop a scar, a place where we are "tougher" than most people. A scar may be less sensitive, but scars, medically speaking, are weaker, less pliable and less able to stretch. This is the same for emotional wounds. What is underneath is still happening and still hurting us. If this rings a bell now but didn't when we went through the questions on emotional trauma, go back and see if they really do apply to you.

Balancing Feeling with Toughness

Of course, there needs to be balance to the Emotional House. It's very healthy to heal what is already there, and a lot of what I have written about deals with this. It's also good to be able to be tough, to build up the muscle to hear unpleasant things, but it needs to be done with awareness.

You can do both things actually, build up a toughness mentally and also have a rich emotional life inside of you. As psychologist Dr. Michael Paul said to me, "The goal is to be like a helicopter: You want to be able to go up and down when you want, not just like a rocket, that only goes up."

Be Aware of Spiritual Bypass!

If something bad has happened to you, and you've said things in your mind like, "It's not that bad...get over it," or "I shouldn't be thinking that" or "don't be angry," you may be doing a spiritual bypass. *A spiritual bypass is a mental defense mechanism used by the brain to avoid feeling something, most likely anger or sadness.* Especially in America, the answer to "How are you?" is not a real answer. People take on a veneer of happiness where it seems that "there are no problems" and "everything is cool." Everything *is* cool... unless it's not. If there are fractured relationships, say, with money, with loved ones, with significant others, if you've had a string of short relationships, if you have had disease and do not know why it's there, chances are very likely there is a "looking inside" that's needed. Usually, in my experience at least, it has to be done in the Emotional House.

Takeaways of the Emotional House

1. Emotional trauma can lead to physical disease if undealt with.

2. By diving deeper into these parts of our history, we can express suppressed feelings and through this expression, we can actually help heal ourselves.

3. We are hard-wired to empathetically experience the events of those around us via mirror neurons. By being aware of who we spend time with and where we spend time, we can help ourselves heal.

EMOTIONAL HOUSE WORKSHEET

Out of the following things discussed in the Emotional House, which one do you feel you need to address the most? (Circle your answer below.)

Issues with father/mother   Anger   Sadness

Unhealed trauma/abuse   Mushrooming   Numbness

What is one change you can make *today* in the area you need to address the most? (Possible changes: journaling, therapy, playing How Do I Feel, playing Free Form Flow)

_____

_____

What stands in your way of making that change?

_____

_____

What can you do to remove that obstacle?

_____

_____

THE SPIRITUAL HOUSE

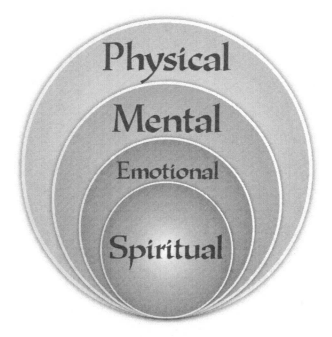

So you've made it this far! Congratulations and thank you. We've gone through almost all the Houses and hopefully you've gotten a good sense that what goes on inside of you affects your health. The first three Houses, Physical, Mental and Emotional, are all for most of us, relatively accessible and acceptable. Even the most cynical among us cannot debate the existence of the body, the mind and the emotions. This comfort-through-proof leads us to more mystical, less externally provable experiences of the

Spiritual House. I don't even think that it's the lack of instant gratification that stops people from making spiritual health part of their daily lives. I think it's lack of awareness that the results we already feel- peace when relaxing quietly, joy when sitting still and seeing a sunset- *are spiritual experiences*. To know that these experiences promote health and to know that it is reproducible is the main reason I (and many others) put spiritual health at the top of the list. We may not always have a healthy body, mind or emotions, but preserving a spiritual sanctuary inside us gives one a refuge when all else is going wrong.

> *"Make your heart a hermitage."*
> - Paramahansa Yogananda,
> Indian yogic master and author

Indeed, simply not being aware that a daily spiritual practice is critical to happiness, let alone health, is probably the reason that so many people in the West don't see its benefits. Consequently, there is unnecessary suffering in the West even in spite of a higher standard of living compared with the East. Los Angeles, where I live, is king when it comes to the spiritual and material dichotomy, where "what really matters" sits ignored right next to "what really doesn't matter." Most of the people strive for more of what doesn't, and when they find that they have a lot of it, they realize how wrong they have been.

"If you realize that you have enough, you are truly rich."
- Lao Tzu, Chinese philosopher

That being said, even in this town I have found plenty of examples of people living a quietly magnificent spiritual life, from the janitor who was so happy I just had to follow him around to watch him, to the burger-flipping guy working his second forty-hour-a-week job and just whistling away. These, unfortunately, are the exceptions. Most of us have so many things that we attach to outside of ourselves for pleasure and comfort, and it only makes sense that we would believe having *more* of these things will only make us happier. By buying more supplements and taking more vitamins, happier and healthier start to look the same. With better medicine, better doctors, better science, we reason that we can probably live forever. This type of thinking can work for years, even decades, but at some point it comes to an end, sometimes because we realize it's all a never-ending cycle, but more likely when something happens to bring us to a new reality (like a disease). My point is, why not choose to integrate a proven methodology *before* things go wrong, so when things do go wrong, you have something powerful and secret inside to rely on? (By the way, this isn't fear speaking: it's prudent self-care and self-love.)

Again, one of the main intentions of this book is to give you tools to make your healing journey a self-directed one. Along the way, I've given you games and evidence to help you show *yourself* how this all can work. This chapter is no different. I'll be giving you evidence to support my assertions and also giving you things to try for yourself. *One main point about the Spiritual House that I want you to consider is that any effort made here can affect the other three Houses, because it lies at the core, affecting everything outside of it.* Every other House can affect other Houses, but only the Spiritual House affects all the others at once. (This is reflected in the diagram you've seen throughout this book: The Spiritual House is the deepest.) Even if your Physical House is so damaged it's hard to change, effort in the Spiritual House has a rippling effect to possibly change either the disease itself, or at the very least, the subjective effect that it has on the mind and emotions.

Secrets to Healing
Within Words We Use for Illness

I was sitting in an airport recently and was looking around me. 90% of the people were unable to sit still, some playing on their phones, and some tapping one leg in rapid fashion. This reminded me of the hidden meanings within two words that are trillion-dollar industries in the US: disease and metastasis.

> *"Stress is the basic cause in 60% of all disease and illness."*
> - American Medical Association

"Disease" we think of as sickness, an illness, something that come from outside of us and invades. In fact, though, the word disease originally meant something much different, and much simpler. As I said in the introduction, I think of the word "disease" simply as a "lack of ease."

The next word that holds a secret meaning is a dreaded word in cancer therapy: *metastasis.* Metastasis means that the cancer has spread beyond the original site, which in studies portends a decreased survival and is much more difficult to get control of, if at all. It originates from the Greek with "meta" meaning beyond and "stasis" meaning stillness. Metastasis: *Beyond stillness.*

For both disease and metastasis, part of the "cure," if you want to call it that, for both things are found right within the words themselves: *ease and stillness.* How do we make these both achievable and reproducible in a crazy, always-on-the-go world? That's what the Spiritual House techniques are all about.

Spiritual Versus Religious

As Gloria Estefan says in her song title, "The Words Get in the Way," this distinction is a good one to elaborate on. Differences in dogma, religious upbringings and forced conceptions of God often get in the way of our own progress towards realizing this presence within us. Throughout this book, I've tried to remove "religious" references as much as I could, to give those of us with strong negative associations around religion a way to open themselves to a deeper personal experience. The goal is to remove the things that can trip us up from finding that peace within, because that's what really is necessary for Spiritual House work. (And by the way, that deeper experience is what *religion* at its core is really is all about: a personal experience of the Divine.)

For those of you who are deeply spiritual, linking that to health might be a no-brainer. For those who have a resistance to spiritual concepts, think of spirituality this way: These are simply scientific techniques, proven through experience for *thousands* of years in the East and more recently through Western studies to improve your stress response, improve your quality of life and make you feel happier.

Every step, if you notice, I've asked you to *try* things, not to believe blindly in them. This is because if they work for you, you will continue doing them. At some point in our lives, we have to look at the Spiritual House and see that its contents have been largely unutilized throughout our lives. It's never been that spiritual effort doesn't work. It's our *conception* of what that House *is* that's been the problem.

Pain Versus Suffering

"Pain is inevitable. Suffering is optional."

- Haruki Murakami,
What I Talk About When I Talk About Running

In the above section, I purposely used the word suffering instead of pain. Some people use the two interchangeably, but for me, there is a subtle but important distinction. From the Merriam-Webster dictionary, pain is "the physical feeling caused by disease, injury, or something that hurts the body." In short, it's a bodily sensation. Suffering, on the other hand, is "the experience of one who is being forced to endure or submit to" something. This encompasses the mental reaction ("I can't believe this is happening to me"), the emotional reaction (anger) and the physical reaction (e.g. Running away). Put another way, pain is a result from the outside, *suffering is what we do to ourselves.*

For most people though, the two are intertwined, so much so that there is no awareness of two separate pro-cesses going on. (No wonder they are used interchangeably!) Pain itself usually doesn't last very long, usually just minutes, and in the case of a bad break (bone or heart) can be days or weeks. Suffering, on the other hand, can last for years and decades, if we so choose to hold onto the pattern. How do we decrease suffering? It's one of those "simple but not easy to do" scenarios: We have to find that space between the pain and suffering. If we can find that space, we will be able to more fully bear the pain without succumbing to the suffering. How do we do that? Meditation.

Meditation, or, If It Sounds Better, Mindfulness-Based Stress Reduction

I once gave a talk to a group of doctors at a hospital and found that people were really receptive to the Houses of Health. They understood the benefit of doing the spiritual work. We even practiced meditation together, and I was really happy. I found out later from one of the attendees that the chaplain of the hospital (who came to the talk and congratulated me after) didn't believe in meditation and wasn't going to promote it, even after all the evidence I presented, because it wasn't acceptable in his paradigm of what spirituality was. This highlights what I said above. Ironically, it isn't usually the scientific part of the mind that has problems, it's the black-and-white irrational mind that cannot accept the word "meditation" because it has religious connotations. So, to get the critical mind off of the word "meditation," I have begun calling it another name, one that has been used often in the scientific literature: mindfulness-based stress reduction or "MBSR."[6] This way it really sounds scientific and not "new agey." For those of you who feel as this chaplain does, please, think of it this way, as Mindfulness-Based Stress Reduction!

---

[6]   MBSR was created by a pioneer in American mind-body movement, Jon Kabat-Zinn.

The Beneficial Effects of Meditation / MBSR

The core of the Spiritual House lies in the practice of meditation. If you've ever tried it, you know its benefits as I list them:

1. Calmness
2. Awareness that our minds are going at a million miles an hour
3. Peace
4. Awareness of suppressed feelings
5. A clarity of purpose on cloudy issues
6. Happiness/Joy
7. Contentment

We have all felt these things when we are calm, maybe while we were sitting on the beach watching the sunset, listening to the waves break. You can see the sunset and the beach environment as calmness-producing, and you might be right. The question is, was it the sunset *itself* that made us feel more peaceful? Or did it give us something to *concentrate on* that was not adding stimulus, so *what was already present inside* could be allowed to surface?

A Task, or a Multitask?

People think of meditation sometimes as a mystical thing, something that "people in Asia do," that makes it seem inaccessible, or worse than that, irrelevant. In fact, nothing could be more relevant for healing than peace of mind, which is what comes with consistent efforts in meditation. In this society, where we are constantly on our cellphones, walking with headphones stuck to our heads across busy streets, talking on Bluetooth in our cars, it seems as if this multitasking must be okay, because, well, "everyone does it." In fact, it's anything but healthy. It's damaging and it's dangerous, and it's almost glorified by our society. The issue is that since it's pervasive and all around us, it influences our behavior. As we learned in the previous section, humans learn best by imitation.

> *"The safest road to hell is the gradual one, the gentle slope, soft underfoot, without sudden turnings, without milestones, without signposts."*
>
> - C.S.Lewis,
> *The Screwtape Letters*

Multitasking increases stress levels,[lxxi] which as we have seen earlier is causative in many diseases. In scientific literature, this particular type of stress is called allostatic load. The more allostatic load we have, the more our brains get depleted and function at a lower efficiency. Plus, as we already learned, increased stressors cause a decrease in immune function. A decrease in immune surveillance increases the risk for disease and cancer recurrence.

Besides the effects it has on our bodies and minds, it has been shown that people who multitask often are *worse* at it than those who don't do it regularly, but they believe that "they are really good multitaskers."[lxxii] So not only is it damaging our health, it's causing us to become delusional!

Learning How To Relax (Again)

As children we could fully get lost in simple things like a sunset, like a bird sitting on a tree. I distinctly remember lying around my bedroom one summer day, waiting for a song to come on the radio, *for a couple hours.* When was the last time you waited two hours for anything? Let alone doing that for two hours and have it feel like *fun?* I know, I know, you don't have time for that, but that's my point. You have to make time for happiness and contentment. Maybe the reason why you remember yourself happier then, is because, well, *you probably were.* You were able to stay in the present moment. Not in the past, not in the future. *Now.*

To get back to that relaxed and contented place is possible, but we have to make a choice to do so. To actually feel more peace and joy in our lives, we need to slow down, to take some time to focus on moments. Meditation can really help bring us back to this childlike state. In stories of saints of all religions, "childlike" is a way these saints are described, and to me part of this characteristic comes from the ability to really be in the moment without regard for the next moment. This process can come in steps though. If you're not ready to close your eyes for a few minutes, learning how to relax by concentrating on a very large object (the sunset or the ocean) or a very small object (a flame on a candle) is a great first step. In fact, in Eastern traditions, it is known that meditation cannot happen until concentration first does. Concentration means focusing the attention on one thing. Sometimes we are naturally able to concentrate and slip into meditation, but speaking from experience, 99% of the time, especially with the multitasking habit of the Western world, concentration is not happening on its own!

(NOTE: When a spontaneous state does arise when you suddenly feel a sense of peace and calmness, try to go with it! It's a gift. Even that to me is difficult; my mind thinks, "Do it later!")

Focusing on an external object that is somewhat stationary is a great way to start. Using a candle is a low cost and low effort starting place- for one, it's easier than driving to the beach to watch a sunset (especially if you live inland). It's a great start because it really lets you see how restless you really are. Sometimes I think I am calm and ready to meditate, but just looking at the candle lets me know I'm not because my eyes will not be able to stay on the lit candle for more than a few seconds! In Sanskrit, one of the oldest languages in the world, this type of concentration technique is called *trataka* and has been practiced for hundreds, if not thousands of years. The fact that it is still around gives some credence to its benefits.

Game #8: Candle Concentration (aka. Trataka)

1. Light a candle, turn off the lights, turn off your cellphones and any distracting devices.

2. Sit in front of the candle in a relaxed position, back straight, palms upturned. (You can either sit on the floor cross-legged or in a chair, whichever is more relaxing and still allows you to keep your spine straight.)

3. Breathe deeply and slowly as you stay focused on the flame.

4. If you get distracted, bring your concentration back to the flame (without judgment!)

5. Time yourself, trying 3 minutes first, then 5 minutes, then increase to 10-15 minutes.

6. Repeat once daily.

Now that we have explored relaxation and concentration with open eyes, it's time to take a look at the closed-eye version.

The First Goal of Meditation

Meditation/MBSR's technical first goal, taking aside its "unprovable" spiritual benefits, is to create a habit of turning inward. Some teachers say the goal is "the absence of thought." My perspective on that is that it's hard for humans to do a negative i.e., to "try not to think." Thus, for me, the first thing is to learn how to observe your breathing. This results in a mind that starts to look inward, or at least, has an awareness of the thoughts that prevent one from looking inward. As we talked about in the Mental House, these thoughts, if they turn negative, barrage the body and cause illness. A mind-body being barraged with thoughts (primarily negative) is given a respite through stillness born of meditation. Through starting a meditation practice, spiritual effort ties right into physical health by making us more aware of our thoughts, and by decreasing allostatic load and stress.

When I suggest meditation to patients, oftentimes I get a blank look, or a look of confusion. It seems to be that certain people feel like it's so foreign to their lives that it can't even be considered. It's too weird, almost. Well, let me give you this personal testimonial: I grew up in Buffalo eating chicken wings and beef sandwiches, watching football and trying to be the biggest winner in everything I did, trying to make myself happy the way the world says to do it. Then out of desperation (when this way didn't work), I tried meditating and it has to be *the single most important change I have made in my life.* Even if you don't believe in it, but are interested in being healthier, I urge you to try it. As the monk who got me hooked said: "I don't want you to believe in it. I want you to try it. If you experiment and it doesn't work, then fine, try something else. But if it works, why would you stop?" I never did!

The only thing I say to people who do want to try it, is to try it for short periods (like seven minutes twice a day) at first. It's like any habit. You have to introduce it slowly for it to take root and not have a negative recoil from your previous restless habits. A friend of mine tried to do *a three-hour* guided meditation the first time he meditated. He made it all the way through, surprisingly, but it was more of a challenge than anything. When I asked him a couple weeks later if he was coming back to meditate at the guided three hour meditation, he replied, "No way! That was way too hard!" Try to start with easy-to-replicate experiences. If you go away wanting more, then that's the right amount of time.

The Evidence for Meditation

Boring! Who wants to read about more research? This section is for you academics because meditation is, in my opinion, a science: the science of stillness. In literature, more and more studies have been accumulating in support of meditation as being good for the body and mind, for healing and overall quality of life. Interestingly, when looking at the data, meditation works both ways: decreasing negative things and increasing positive things. It really all depends on how the researchers wanted to look at the data. In a mental framing sense, this is very interesting: Is decreasing your negatives the same as increasing your positives? Some traditions focus on *removing* attachments that will make you suffer, like Buddhism for example, where the goal is absence of suffering. Some focus on the positive, connecting only with that which is love and good, Bhakti Yoga, for example. It seems to me that the best path is (surprise!) doing both, removing negatives and highlighting positives.

In a review[lxxiii] of 47 studies done by Goyal et.al., it was found that meditation significantly[lxxiv] decreased anxiety, depression and pain. These 47 studies included all diseases, including cancer. If you're reading this and have been through cancer treatment, you know that anxiety, depression, and pain are big factors in going through and recovering from treatment. In these studies looked at in the review, 30-40 minutes a day was the average amount of meditation done.

There have been studies looking at meditation in cancer patients only. From my review, they mostly have used the Buddhist-derived technique mentioned earlier, mindfulness-based stress reduction (MBSR) as taught by Jon Kabat-Zinn, 90 minutes once a week for eight weeks with a one-day retreat at the end. Because Kabat-Zinn emphasized the biological and not theological aspects of meditation, it became more accepted to study. One of the larger studies, by Branstrom et.al., [lxxv]showed a benefit in perceived stress (anxiety) and posttraumatic-type symptoms. There will be more and more of this research coming out, hopefully with more "marketing" behind them to put it out into the minds of the public. If you're getting excited about the possibilities of what meditation can do for you, then *you* will be the way it spreads. Influencing your friends by your own positive changes is the most impactful and lasting way you improve your world.

"Be the change you want to see in the world."
-Mahatma Gandhi

How the Brain and Body Changes with Meditation

Most of the studies above are about how a person's experience changes with meditation. There is also very tantalizing evidence when looking directly at the brain and the body's biochemistry. When examining MRIs of the brain, researchers found that the brain of longtime meditators actually have a different brain structure than those of people who do not meditate. They demonstrate thicker insular, amygdala, and frontal cortex areas.[lxxvi] These areas are associated with emotions and emotional response. What does a thicker area mean? It means these areas are more developed, meaning those people are more able to experience emotion and emotional events in a healthier, less traumatic way. It's like going to the gym: meditation trains the brain like a muscle. It's just that the weights are different.

It has been found that the stress hormones floating around the body in cancer patients who took a meditation course were lower as well.[lxxvii] Stress hormones, including cortisol, were found to be lower one year after taking an eight-week course. This is significant because cortisol has an important role in causing disease through chronic inflammation. These stress hormones have a role in repairing injury, which is a good thing, but when they are active without an actual physical injury- being increased by life stress- they can themselves *cause* disease, i.e., cancer. There is also emerging evidence that prolonged exposure to stress affects your DNA health, with studies showing it decreases telomere length (which we talked about earlier being a marker for healthy DNA replication). A study done in 2010 showed that people taking a 3-month meditation retreat had significantly more telomerase activity (telo-merase is active when making more telomeres) after the meditation retreat[lxxviii] than those who were stuck on a wait list. (Don't worry, the wait list people got to go later!)

Changing Your Neural Grooves

*"You cannot solve a problem with the same
mind that created it."*

- Albert Einstein

Not only does meditation have *direct* changes to the brain and body, it also sets the stage for change *indirectly* by allowing the brain to rewire itself. Dr. Herbert Benson, a leader in mind-body medicine from Harvard University who has authored over 200 scientific papers and 11 books, spent his life researching this effect. He says, "Through meditation... you can set the stage for important mind and habit-altering brain change."[lxxix] Dr. Stephen Smith, a leading researcher in brain anatomy and synaptic connections at Stanford University, estimates that there are over 200 billion neurons in the brain, with 125 trillion synaptic connections in the cerebral cortex alone. Each neuron has the potential to interact with *hundreds* of other neurons via thousands of synapses, each synapse has hundreds of switches.[lxxx] That's a staggering number of interwoven networks.

These networks work like roads through a city, if the city were a brain. If a thought were a car, cars (mental thoughts) theoretically can travel through the city on all the roads (neural pathways). However, as people who drive every day, you know that there are "favorite" routes (thought patterns) that get driven more. When rush hour comes (stress), these pathways get overloaded and over time they get used even when there are possibly better ways to go, simply because *that's the way we've always gone.* Also, what happens when we drive these roads without repair? Potholes (obsessive and destructive mental thoughts)!

What does all this information mean for our journey of healing? By knowing there are pathways, perhaps *unlimited* numbers of pathways, we can choose to find new ways to think and respond, perhaps ways that are better than the ways we have always thought or responded. In addition to the games we have learned in the Mental House (Poise and The Others) that help us think new thoughts in the same situations, meditation adds the foundation for mental rewiring to take place, by allowing a balancing of the left and right hemispheres and opening new thought possibilities. In our car analogy, meditation is like a navigation app, like Waze or Google Maps, which gives us a new possibility on how to get home faster with less frustration. The catch? We have to remember to *look* at the map program before we go, i.e., *to meditate* before making the same old mistakes.

How Much Meditation Do I Have to Do?

This is a common question I get, and the answer that I've come to may surprise you: *7 minutes twice a day.* There are a couple reasons why I give this number and both reasons are practical. One is that some studies that demonstrated an improvement using meditation utilized 90 minutes a week as their meditation routine. Ninety minutes a week breaks down to just over 6 minutes twice a day. The second reason why I say to do it twice a day is to make it a habit: It establishes a routine, which if you continue doing it will provide long-term benefits. It sounds doable, right? I have been recommending this to my patients who are interested, and it seems to be catching on. If you do 98 minutes each week (7 minutes x 2 x 7 days) after a whole year you'll have done 5096 minutes, or 84 hours of meditation!

Game #9: 7 Minute Meditation

1. Find a timer (most phones have a timer function now!). Set it for 7 minutes.

2. Find a quiet spot.

3. Assume an upright posture: Sit on a chair, feet flat on the floor, palms open, back straight (away from the back of the chair), chin horizontal to the floor, eyes closed, eyes upturned without tension. (If you can sit on the ground, cross-legged with your back straight without tension, that works.)

4. Take three deep breaths, inhaling and exhaling slowly. Release any tense areas during these breaths.

5. After the third breath, let yourself breathe naturally.

6. Let any thoughts come through your mind, and let them exit. Do not judge.

7. If the mind is very active, think on the inhale: "Peace," and think on the exhale "Tension."

8. When you hear the timer go off, deeply inhale once and slowly open your eyes.

***If you want a guided version, you may use the 7 Minute Meditation Video on YouTube that I uploaded.
(Search "Roy Vongtama Seven Minute Meditation.")

Committing to Your Practice

In martial arts, when one makes a commitment, it is called "putting iron around it." This means it is not to be violated for any reason. You and I both know full well the difficulty in getting something started, and we both know how even more difficult it is to keep something going. By putting mental "iron" around your meditation practice, you are vowing to do it, no matter what happens, no matter how busy you get. After all, it's only 7 minutes!

Final Thoughts on Meditation

I've tried to give you a simple way to approach meditation, in addition to the benefits you might accrue by doing it. There are a bunch of free apps on your phone that you can try that can guide you into a meditation habit. I'm not saying it won't be hard to latch onto, but as I said before, sticking to a meditation habit was the single most important thing I have done in the last fifteen years. Of course, it's not going to be easy, but nothing worth doing is easy, is it?

Game #10: What is Missing Now?

Objective: A koan is a Zen riddle that is designed to result in you looking inward. "What is missing now?" is a highly effective koan. It instinctively causes you to really consider the question's answer. At the risk of totally ruining the simplicity of the koan, let's break it down.

How to Play: Ask yourself, "What's missing right now?" Consider the answers that arise.

When to play: When you feel discontented about a situation in your life. I use this question whenever I get "that feeling" that I should be more successful or somewhere different or with someone different. Those are ideas I have imposed upon myself and cause me to feel scarcity. Those questions (Why me? What about me?) can be great things to introspect on in a controlled way, but usually they are running in our heads without permission.

Notes: "What is missing now?" really is asking "what is missing that is allowing you to remain unhappy in this very moment?" And the answer is: *Feeling* like something is missing. Unless you are in acute pain, 99% of the time the answer is, in this *very* moment, nothing is missing. Our minds may want more money, want "things to be different," wish that someone might not have left our lives, wished that we not lost our job, et cetera, but in reality, as you sit here reading this line, *nothing is missing but our ability to recognize that we are complete.* Simply the realization that all is well right now can bring that instant peace to us. This is mindfulness in an instant. Take control back and ask yourself: *What is missing now?*

The Value of Introspection

When we buy a car, it goes through a mandatory inspection. Periodically it has to pass inspections- for brakes, smog, oil, and every week or so it gets a car wash. Even daily, our cars are always self-checking: they monitor for low fuel, low wiper fluid, engine heat, low coolant, low tire pressure, etc. Ironically, we have made it so our cars are checked much more frequently than our own selves!

This self-inspection process is just as critical for us as human beings. Introspection means to take a look inside oneself, hopefully as objectively as our car's sensors do. When I say "objectively," I mean without blame or judgment. Like our cars, the best way is to do a daily shorter version and a more comprehensive yearly one.

How important is introspection? In the Bhagavad Gita, the Hindu equivalent of the Bible, *the very first line* is about introspection. Bhagavan Krishna asks his disciple Arjuna that very question: "How did you fare today on the battleground?" Metaphysically it means not just on the battlefield of daily life, but in your mind and heart as well. That is the question we must ask at the end of the day, as objectively as possible, without judgment or rationalization.

For daily introspection, I would recommend it before bed, after your nightly meditation (if you are incorporating meditation). I am a big proponent of writing it down. Why? It gets it out of conception (your head) and into the real world. Every night, or every few nights at least, I take out my journal and really check in with myself, "How did today go?" This process is an amazingly effective one. Sometimes there are things that were unprocessed, "I'll deal with that later" type-stuff that I had forgotten, and it resurfaces at that point. You'll also find that if you start meditating, that these thoughts will start to surface and you'll find that the introspection period is a good time to process them.

It doesn't have to be a long journaling period. Most of mine take 5-10 minutes max. Why not longer? Like meditation, it shouldn't become a stress, rather it should be stress relief. I look forward to it now, it feels like closure to the day.

> *"Always leave 'em wanting more."*
> -Showbiz maxim

Of course, if it's necessary, take a longer period to really unravel a clouded situation. Clarity is mostly all you need to return to calmness. Your body, mind and soul will thank you for it.

Gratitude Versus Desires

"Your attitude, not your aptitude, determines your altitude."
- Zig Ziglar,
motivational speaker

"Gratitude is the attitude."
-unknown

"Resentment cannot enter a grateful heart."
-paraphrased from
an unknown monk

One of the main spiritual concepts I want to convey about health is the idea of gratitude as an attitude. I had a conversation with a friend recently and we were talking about visualization. She had been reading about the power of using visualizations to materialize things that she really wanted in this life. I thought that was great for her and was very encouraging, especially as she felt she wasn't worthy of having her dreams materialize. This was important for her growth. If you have this feeling, then all the better to see yourself with those things you never thought you could have.

Later, after I left this friend, I realized I don't focus on the things that I want anymore. The metaphysical reason is because I have found the Universe brings to you more of *what you already are, not what you want to be.* The more you appreciate and validate inside of you what things already are in your life, the more it will be part of your consciousness, the more it will come to you. This isn't to say that desiring things is wrong. It's really that appreciating what you already have will allow you to feel happy with what is there, and what comes after is icing on the cake. A monk I know says, "You cannot give of your own half-full cup. When your cup runs over, you can give the overflow to others." It's like the car analogy from above. A lot of us who get sick have had the "check engine" light on for months, if not years. The big pivot point is to realize that *you* come first, and secondly, to realize that being grateful really is the secret. If you don't have the big things, don't worry, give thanks for the small things.

How many stories have you heard of people who have "risen to the top" and been completely miserable, to the point where they have taken their own lives or have tried to? It's too many to mention names. We hear about it so much nowadays, we just shake our heads and don't really dissect why it happens. But why does it happen? It happens at a basic level because it's very easy to get tricked by the world into thinking that the trappings of happiness we hold in our heads *are the same thing as happiness.* And really, they are just that, trappings. *They trap us into thinking they are necessary for happiness.*

In fact, the amassing of material "evidence" of success and prosperity can be a sign of true internal prosperity OR a spotlight of deep scarcity. In the first case, the energy around the person is one of gratitude and abundance, and in the second, the energy is one of loneliness, anxiety and scarcity. So it's so important to cultivate this gratitude. How do you develop an attitude of gratitude? Start by acknowledging what's already there.

The Laws of Motion Applied to Gratitude

I said above that gratitude is a metaphysical concept, and it is, but it is also rooted in the natural laws that are visible around us. The third law of motion is, "Every action has an equal and opposite reaction." This is not just about objects and Sir Isaac Newton. Since it is a Law that applies to this world, it applies also to your actions and your thoughts! If you are thinking positive thoughts of gratitude and valuing the things that surround you, more of those things will come to you. The first law of motion is "An object in motion stays in motion, an object at rest stays at rest." Translated in terms of gratitude, if you are moving forward in a positive way in your mind, it will be easier to stay in that motion. If you decide to stay stuck, then that's also where you will be. The *inertia* will keep you stuck and it is what makes it really hard to start a new habit, because in that area of your life, you've been 'at rest' for a long time.

Game #11: Five Stars a Day

Introspection, once you get good at it, can really help you see what's going well and what's not. Unfortunately, the *critical* eye is the easier one to hone in with, usually with the good intention of improving yourself. However, I have a newsflash for you: you're not ever going to be perfect. So only looking at what you can improve isn't really balanced and for sure it's not healthy. After coaching with two success consultants, Craig Marshall and Andrew Papageorge, I started implementing this gratitude practice.

1. Get a journal. (It never leaves your bedside. I use a black 'composition book.')

2. Make five stars on five separate lines.

3. Write down five great moments of your day.

4. Re-experience these five events.

Some days you find ten things, and there are ten stars, and those are amazing days. More often though, it can be an effort to find five! Here's the thing though: it can be anything that felt good during the day for you to star: The simple experience of watching a hummingbird can be a "starred" event. Sometimes it's that I watched an episode of my favorite show. Sometimes it's that I had a great experience in meditation. Some nights, after a hard day, when you'd think I'd just want to go to sleep and forget the day, I still pull out my journal because of the great habit I developed. Other nights I get excited because I want to see what actually went well, and because I make a habit out of looking for good things, I seem to find them.

REMINDER NOTE for Step 4: Re-experiencing these events: This practice is significantly enhanced when one is able to savor these events *again*. Why? As I stated earlier, the body and mind do not know the difference between a replay of an old event and a brand new one if you are fully present in it.

SPIRITUAL HOUSE WORKSHEET

Out of the following things discussed in the Spiritual House, which one do you feel might help you the most?   (Circle)

Going into Nature   Meditation/MBSR

Trataka (Candle concentration)

Are you willing to try one of those things today?

_____

_____

What stands in your way of making that change?

_____

_____

What can you do to remove that obstacle?

_____

_____

FINAL THOUGHTS

I hope this book has brought you some new perspectives, things that you can take with you on your healing journey.

I have one more story to share:

A former cancer patient, Chris, related to me the experience he had when he had Hodgkin's lymphoma at the age of 21. He mentioned to me, "You can learn a lot in the waiting room." I asked him what he meant. He described his inner world at the age of 21 as, "This sucks, but it's gonna be over and then I'll be back partying and studying again." He was there for his last chemotherapy session and across from him sat an elderly couple holding hands. They inquired, "Is this your last treatment?" He nodded. "Is this yours?" They smiled, "Well..." pausing for a moment. "He's had a good run. We're going to let it ride after this meeting."

This stopped him in his tracks. What they meant, he found out, was that the elderly man's cancer was incurable, and that the treatment wasn't working anymore, and that they were going to let nature take its course. C.W. said, "It changed my entire life. I saw everything differently after that. What I thought wasn't going to define me (the cancer) became the *reason* for me realizing the world isn't all about *me*. I began to have that gratitude."

Knowing him as a person and a friend, I could feel the truth in him, that the experience gives him a compassionate perspective even to this day. This is a great story, but I have also heard many where the change in perspective *hasn't* lasted, where the experience was, and continues to be, another example of how they have been victimized by life. So really, what I am saying is this: It's a choice. And spiritually and truthfully, what we must decide is that our challenges, diseases included, can be gifts.

After spending over seven years and hundreds of hours researching and writing this book, I reflected on what would make it a success. The fact that you are reading this means it affected you enough to finish it. However, for me that's not enough. If I had one hope, it would be that I have inspired you to change at least one thing *permanently* in your life for the better. If you can take responsibility, take ownership, even for one small thing, and change that thing into a lasting habit, then this book, *Healing Before You're Cured,* will be a success. Moreover, if you can choose to listen to the healing message disease can contain, and have gratitude daily for that enlarged perspective, instead of being the victim, *you* become the living proof that you can be healed, not just cured.

SPECIAL THANKS

To all the patients and friends who asked questions and inspired me to write this book, Mom and Dad for pushing me to be the best I can be, Dan and Melissa for being supportive, Mei Ling Moore and Dan Vongtama for giving notes and proofreading, Joshua Galitsky and Steven Friedlander for editing parts of the book, Meena Makhijani for her encouragement and love, Samira Jeihooni for reading and giving notes, Dr. Guy Juillard for pushing me to finish the book and through his tremendous example, God and Guru for their constant guidance.

Like what you read? Want more? Access Dr. Vongtama's new articles and videos on Mind-Body Medicine by visiting www.MDRoy.com.

FINAL WORKSHEET

What House do you feel you need to address the most?

_____

Why?

_____

_____

What *one* change can you commit to in this House, on a daily basis, for *ten weeks*? (Remember research shows 10 weeks is the cutoff point for ingraining a new habit.)

Fill in this sentence and sign it:

I, _____, commit to
_____ for ten
weeks. I know it will be for my highest good.

_____
(signature)

BIBLIOGRAPHY

In this bibliography, I have endeavored to make it user friendly. Oftentimes they are totally useless as only people with subscriptions to academic journals can access the sources. If I was able to include a website or link to it, I have!

---

[i] Siegel RL, Miller KD, Jemal A. Cancer statistics, 2015. CA Cancer J Clin. 2015 Jan-Feb; 65(1):5-29. doi: 10.3322/caac.21254. Epub 2015 Jan 5.

[ii] Beckett, Samuel. *Worstward Ho.* New York: Grove Press, 1983.

[iii] Willcox BJ, Willcox DC, et. Al. Caloric restriction, the traditional Okinawan diet, and healthy aging: the diet of the world's longest-lived people and its potential impact on morbidity and life span. *Annals of the New York Academy of Science.* 2007 Oct;1114:434-55

[iv] Teo K, Lear S, Islam S, et.al. Prevalence of a Healthy

Lifestyle Among Individuals With Cardiovascular Disease in High-, Middle- and Low-Income Countries The Prospective Urban Rural Epidemiology (PURE) Study. *JAMA.* 2013;309(15):1613–1621.

[v] Overton, Patrick. *The leaning tree.* Bethany Press. 1975

[vi] Dunn GP, Old LJ, Schreiber RD. The three Es of cancer immunoediting. Annu Rev Immunol. 2004;22:329-60. Review.

[vii] Dolan DE, Gupta S. PD-1 pathway inhibitors: changing the landscape of cancer immunotherapy. Cancer Control. 2014 Jul;21(3):231-7. Review.

[viii] McCoy KD, Le Gros G. The role of CTLA-4 in the regulation of T cell immune responses. Immunol Cell Biol. 1999 Feb;77(1):1-10. Review.

[ix] Warburton DER, Nicol CW, Bredin SSD. Health benefits of physical activity: the evidence. *CMAJ : Canadian Medical Association Journal.* 2006;174(6):801-809. doi:10.1503/cmaj.051351.

[x] Lally P, van Jaarsveld CHM, Potts HWW, Wardle J. How are habits formed: modelling habit formation in the real world. Euro J Soc Psychol. 2010;40:998–1009.

[xi] Soret S, et.al. *Climate change mitigation and health effects of varied dietary patterns in real-life settings throughout North America.* Am J Clin Nutr. 2014 Jul;100 Suppl 1:490S-5S. doi: 10.3945/ajcn.113.071589. Epub 2014 Jun 4. PubMed PMID: 24898230.

[xii] www.who.int   or type "WHO" and "sugar recommendation" into Google.

[xiii] Yang Q. Gain weight by "going diet?" Artificial sweeteners and the neurobiology of sugar cravings: Neuroscience 2010. *The Yale Journal of Biology and Medicine.* 2010;83(2):101-108.

[xiv] Cuatrecasas P, Lockwood DH, Caldwell JR. Lactase deficiency in the adult: a common occurrence. *Lancet.* 1965;1:14-18.

[xv] Looker AC, Johnston CC, Wahner HW, et al. Prevalence of low femoral bone density in older U.S. women from NHANES III. *J Bone and Mineral Research.* 1995;10:796-802.

[xvi] Chan JM, Stampfer MJ, Ma J, Gann PH, Gaziano JM, Giovannucci E. Dairy products, calcium, and prostate cancer risk in the Physicians' Health Study. *Am J Clin Nutr.* 2001;74:549-554.

xvii Larsson SC, Orsini N, Wolk A. Milk, milk products and lactose intake and ovarian cancer risk: a meta-analysis of epidemiological studies. *Int J Cancer*. 2006;118(2):431-441.

xviii Levine et.al. Low Protein Intake Is Associated with a Major Reduction in IGF-1, Cancer, and Overall Mortality in the 65 and Younger but Not Older Population. Cell Metabolism, Volume 19, Issue 3, 407-417, 4 March 2014

xix Cross AJ, Leitzmann MF, Gail MH, Hollenbeck AR, Schatzkin A, Sinha R (2007) A Prospective Study of Red and Processed Meat Intake in Relation to Cancer Risk. PLoS Med4(12): e325. https://doi.org/10.1371/journal.pmed.0040325

xv Fraser et.al. Associations between diet and cancer, ischemic heart disease, and all-cause mortality in non-Hispanic white California Seventh-day Adventists American Journal of Clinical Nutrition 1999 70: 532s-538s

xxi http://www.choosemyplate.gov/MyPlate

xxii CDC.gov 2013-2014 statistics. Probably even higher now.

xxiii Bianchini F, Kaaks R, Vainio H. Overweight, obesity, and cancer risk. Lancet Oncol. 2002 Sep;3(9):565-74.

Review.

[xxiv] Basen-Engquist, K. & Chang, *Obesity and Cancer Risk, Recent Review and Evidence* M. Curr Oncol Rep (2011) 13: 71.

[xxv] Roberts, D.L. et.al. *Biological Mechanisms Linking Obesity and Cancer Risk: New Perspectives.* Annual Review of Medicine 2010 61:1, 301-316

[xxvi] Guarner F, Schaafsma GJ (1998): Probiotics. Int J Food Microbiol, 39: 237-238.

[xxvii] Sender R, Fuchs S, Milo R (2016) *Revised Estimates for the Number of Human and Bacteria Cells in the Body.* PLoS Biol14(8): e1002533. https://doi.org/10.1371/journal.pbio.1002533

[xxviii] McFarland L.V. (2006) Meta-analysis of probiotics for the prevention of antibiotic associated diarrhea and the treatment of Clostridium difficile disease. Am J Gastroenterol 101: 812–822

[xxix] Bhatt AP, Redinbo MR, Bultman SJ. The role of the microbiome in cancer development and therapy. CA Cancer J Clin. 2017 Jul 8;67(4):326-344. doi: 10.3322/caac.21398. Epub 2017 May 8. Review. PubMed PMID: 28481406

[xxx]*Health and Nutritional Properties of Probiotics in Food including Powder Milk with Live Lactic Acid Bacteria*, World Health Organization Report 2001. http://www.who.int/foodsafety/publications/fs_management/en/probiotics.pdf

[xxxi] Elazab, N.; Mendy, A.; Gasana, J.; Vieira, E. R.; Quizon, A.; Forno, E. (2013). "Probiotic Administration in Early Life, Atopy, and Asthma: A Meta-analysis of Clinical Trials". *Pediatrics* **132** (3): e666–76.

[xxxii] Saikali, J., Picard, C., Freitas, M., Holt, P. (2004). Fermented Milks, Probiotic Cultures, and Colon Cancer. Nutrition and Cancer. 49(1): 14-24

[xxxiii] Viaud, S. et.al. The Intestinal Microbiota Modulates the Anticancer Immune Effects of Cyclophosphamide. Science 22 November 2013: Vol. 342 no. 6161 pp. 971-976

[xxxiv] Ridaura, VK. Et.al. Gut *Microbiota from Twins Discordant for Obesity Modulate Metabolism in Mice.*Science 6 September 2013: Vol. 341 no. 6150
[xxxv] Alcock J, Maley CC, Aktipis CA. Is eating behavior manipulated by the gastrointestinal microbiota? Evolutionary pressures and potential mechanisms. Bioessays. 2014 Oct;36(10):940-9. doi:

10.1002/bies.201400071. Epub 2014 Aug 8. Review.

xxxvi Collins, S. The Intestinal Microbiota Affect Central Levels of Brain-Derived Neurotropic Factor and Behavior in Mice. Volume 141, Issue 2 , Pages 599-609.e3, August 2011

xxxvii Hublin C, Partinen M, Koskenvuo M, Kaprio J. Sleep and mortality: a population-based 22-year follow-up study. Sleep. 2007 Oct 1;30(10):1245-53.Patel SR, Ayas NT, Malhotra MR, White DP, Schernhammer ES, Speizer FE, Stampfer MJ, Hu FB. A prospective study of sleep duration and mortality risk in women. Sleep. 2004 May 1;27(3):440-4.

xxxviii Porkka-Heiskanen T. 1999. Adenosine in sleep and wakefulness. Annals of Medicine. 31:125-129.

xxxix Besedovsky L., Lange, T., Born, J Sleep and immune function. Pflugers Arch. 2012 January; 463(1): 121–137.

xl Sigurdson K, Ayas N. 2007. The public health and safety consequences of sleep disorders. Canadian J Physiol Pharmacol. 85:179-183.
http://www.mdanderson.org/newsroom/news-releases/2012/depression-shortened-telomeres-increase-

mortality-in-bladder-cancer-patients.html

xli *Food, Nutrition, Physical Activity and the Prevention of Cancer.* American Institute for Cancer Research, 2007. An excellent FREE resource available at www.dietandcancerreport.org

xlii Effect of physical activity on cognitive function in older adults at risk for Alzheimer disease: a randomized trial. JAMA 2009 Jan 21;301(3):276 Lautenschlager NT et al.

xliii http://www.cancer.gov/cancertopics/factsheet/Risk/obesity

xliv Crockett SD, et.al. Calcium and vitamin D supplementation and increased risk of serrated polyps: results from a randomised clinical trial. Gut. 2018 Mar 1. pii: gutjnl-2017-315242. doi: 10.1136/gutjnl-2017-315242.

xlv Holick, Michael F. *The Vitamin D Solution: A Three Step Strategy to Cure Our Most Common Health Problem.* Penguin Press 2010.

xlvi Schernhammer, E. S. *et al.* Rotating night shifts and risk of breast cancer in women participating in the nurses' health study. *J. Natl Cancer Inst.* 93, 1563–1568 (2001).

xlvii Chevalier, G, et.al. *The effect of earthing (grounding) on human physiology*. European Biology Magazine 2006;2(1): 600-621 (out of print but full paper available online. Search Google!)

xlviii Chevalier, G. Et.al. *Earthing (Grounding) the Human Body Reduces Blood Viscosity—a Major Factor in Cardiovascular Disease*. The Journal of Alternative and Complementary Medicine, Vol 19: 2, 2013 (102–110) (available for free online. Search Title in Google!)

xlix Fredrickson, B. L., & Losada, M. F. (2005). Positive affect and complex dynamics of human flourishing. American Psychologist, 60, 678-686.

li Segerstrom SC, Taylor SE, Kemeny ME, Fahey JL. Optimism is associated with mood, coping, and immune change in response to stress. J Pers Social Psychol. 1998;74:1646–1655.

lii Lipton, B. *The Biology of Belief: Unleashing the Power of Consciousness, Matter & Miracles*. Hay House. 2006.

liii Wolkowitz O.M. *Leukocyte telomere length in major depression: correlations with chronicity,inflammation and oxidative stress--preliminary findings*. PLoS One. 2011 Mar 23;6(3):e17837

[liv] F. W. Lung, N. C. Chen, and B. C. Shu, *Genetic pathway of major depressive disorder in shortening telomeric length*, Psychiatric Genetics, vol. 17, no. 3, pp. 195–199, 2007.

[lv] Epel E,et.al. *Can meditation slow rate of cellular aging? Cognitive stress, mindfulness, and telomeres.* Ann NY Acad Sci. 2009 Aug;1172:34-53.

[lvi] Seligman, Martin. *Learned Optimism: How to Change Your Mind and Your Life* 1991 New York: Knopf. (Paperback reprint edition, Penguin Books, 1998; reissue edition, Free Press, 1998). Also *Flourish: A Visionary New Understanding of Happiness and Well-being.* New York: Free Press 2011.

[lvii] Anthony D. Mancini, et.al. *Stepping Off the Hedonic Treadmill Individual Differences in Response to Major Life Events,* Journal of Individual Differences 2011; Vol. 32(3):144–152

[lviii] Rosenzweig P, Brohier S, Zipfel A. The placebo effect in healthy volunteers: influence of experimental conditions on the adverse events profile during phase I studies. Clin Pharmacol Ther 1993;54:578-83.

[lix] Shalev I, et.al. *Exposure to violence during childhood is*

associated with telomere erosion from 5 to 10 years of age: a longitudinal study. Mol Psychiatry. 2013 May;18(5):576-81.

lx *Relationship of Childhood Abuse and Household Dysfunction to Many of the Leading Causes of Death in Adults.* Felitti, Vincent J et al. American Journal of Preventive Medicine , Volume 14 , Issue 4 , 245 – 258

lxi Brown MJ, Thacker LR, Cohen SA. *Association between Adverse Childhood Experiences and Diagnosis of Cancer.* Vinciguerra M, ed. *PLoS ONE.* 2013;8(6):e65524. doi:10.1371/journal.pone.0065524.

lxii Lillberg K, et.al. Stressful life events and risk of breast cancer in 10,808 women: a cohort study. American Journal of Epidemiology. 2003;157:415–423.

lxiii First Marriages in the United States: Data From the 2006–2010 National Survey of Family Growth by Casey E. Copen, Ph.D.; Kimberly Daniels, Ph.D.; Jonathan Vespa, Ph.D.; and William D. Mosher, Ph.D., Division of Vital Statistics. National Health Statistics Reports Number 49. March 22, 2012.

[lxiv] Taillieu TL,et.al. *Childhood emotional maltreatment and mental disorders: Results from a nationally representative adult sample from the United States.* Child Abuse Negl. 2016 Sep;59:1-12.

[lxv] Cloitre M, Garvert DW, Weiss B, Carlson EB, Bryant RA. Distinguishing PTSD, Complex PTSD, and Borderline Personality Disorder: A latent class analysis. Eur J Psychotraumatol. 2014 Sep 15;5.

[lxvi] Gibran, Kahlil. *The Prophet.* Alfred A. Knopf. HARDCOVER edition.1972.

[lxvii] The Diagnostic and Statistical Manual used by psychologists for defining disorders and mental illness. Currently they are in version 5, or, "DSM-5".

[lxviii] Shedler, Jonathan. *Efficacy of Psychodynamic Therapy* The American psychologist 2010 Feb-Mar;65(2):98-109 Available to read online. Search title in Google!

[lxix] Abbass, A., Kisely, S. & Kroenke, K (2009). Short-Term Psychodynamic Psychotherapy for Somatic Disorders: Systematic Review and Meta-Analysis of Clinical Trials. Psychotherapy and Psychosomatics, 78, 265-274.

[lxx] Rizzolatti G, Craighero L. The mirror-neuron system. Annu Rev Neurosci. 2004;27:169-92. Review.

lxxi McEwen, Bruce S. "Stress, adaptation, and disease: Allostasis and allostatic load." *Annals of the New York Academy of Sciences* 840.1 (1998): 33-44.

lxxii Executive Control of Cognitive Processes in Task Switching. Journal of Experimental Psychology: Human Perception and Performance, 27(4), 763-797. Kieras, D. E., Meyer, D. E., Ballas, J. A., & Lauber, E. J. (2001)

lxxiii Madhav G. et.al. *Meditation Programs for Psychological Stress and Well-being.* JAMA Internal Medicine, 2014;174(3):357-368

lxxiv When a study is found to be "significant," they are talking about statistically significant. What does this mean? It means that the result is very unlikely due to chance. Sometimes studies are not statistically significant, but even that doesn't mean that the treatment isn't effective. It just may mean that particular study didn't have enough subjects or wasn't designed correctly.

lxxv Bränström R, Kvillemo P, Brandberg Y, Moskowitz JT. Self-report mindfulness as a mediator of psychological well-being in a stress reduction intervention for cancer patients--a randomized study. Ann Behav Med. 2010 May;39(2):151-61.

lxxvi Murakami H, Nakao T, Matsunaga M, Kasuya Y, Shinoda J, et al. (2012) The Structure of Mindful Brain. PLoS ONE 7(9): e46377. doi:10.1371/journal.pone.0046377 (full text available online!!)

lxxvii Carlson LE, Speca M, Faris P, Patel KD. One year pre-post intervention follow-up of psychological, immune, endocrine and blood pressure outcomes of mindfulness-based stress reduction (MBSR) in breast and prostate cancer outpatients. Brain Behav Immun. 2007 Nov;21(8):1038-49. Epub 2007 May 22.

lxxviii Jacobs TL et.al. *Intensive meditation training, immune cell telomerase activity, and psychological mediators.* Psychoneuroendocrinology. 2011 Jun;36(5):664-81. doi: 10.1016/j.psyneuen.2010.09.010. Epub 2010 Oct 29

lxxix Benson, Herbert. *Your Maximum Mind.* New York: Random House, 1987.

lxxx Micheva, Kristina D. et al. Single-Synapse Analysis of a Diverse Synapse Population: Proteomic Imaging Methods and Markers. Neuron , Volume 68 , Issue 4 , 639 - 653

Made in the USA
San Bernardino, CA
29 July 2019